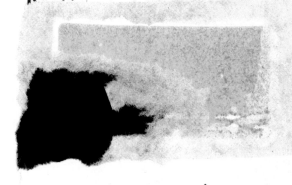

withdrawn from
stock 16|4|24

8·95

Pocket Examiner in
Psychiatry

Patrick McKeon MD MRCPI MRCPsych
Clinical Teacher, University of Dublin; Consultant
Psychiatrist, St Patrick's Hospital, Dublin

Eilish Gilvarry MRCPsych MRCGP DCH DObs
Senior Registrar in Psychiatry, Parkwood House, St
Nicholas's Hospital, Gosforth, Newcastle-upon-Tyne

Churchill Livingstone

EDINBURGH LONDON MELBOURNE AND NEW YORK 1988

CHURCHILL LIVINGSTONE
Medical Division of Longman Group UK Limited

Distributed in the United States of America by Churchill
Livingstone Inc., 1560 Broadway, New York, N.Y. 10036,
and by associated companies, branches and representatives
throughout the world.

First published 1988

ISBN 0-443-03711-6

British Library Cataloguing in Publication Data
McKeon, Patrick
    Pocket examiner in psychiatry
    1. Psychiatry—Problems, exercises, etc.
    I. Title   II. Gilvarry, Eilish
    616.89′0076   RC457

Library of Congress Cataloging in Publication Data
McKeon, Patrick.
    Pocket examiner in psychiatry/Patrick McKeon, Eilish
    Gilvarry.
    Includes index.
    ISBN 0-443-03711-6
    1. Psychiatry—Examinations, questions, etc. I. Gilvarry,
    Eilish.   II. Title.
    [DNLM: 1. Psychiatry — examination questions.
    WM 18 M478p]
    RC457.M395 1988
    616.89′0076—dc19

Produced by Longman Singapore Publishers (Pte) Ltd.
Printed in Singapore

Preface

'Uncertainty' and 'immediacy' are the two words that probably best describe the particular difficulties that confront candidates in all examinations. Uncertainty about what topic the examiner may light upon has its own dread, knowing that the range of enquiry may be much more focused than in an essay or multiple choice examination question and may reflect the personal interest of the examiner. The need for an immediate response to the examiner's question is equally daunting and doubly so when one considers the 'uncertainty' factor.

The aim of this book is to prepare the candidate for oral examinations by presenting a comprehensive range of challenging questions with answers in random order. While the compilation is primarily intended for MRCPsych examination candidates, final year medical students and postgraduate doctors wishing to update their knowledge will find it a helpful teaching aid. The questions should be answered aloud, preferably to a colleague, before the text answer is read. Each answer gives a detailed resume of the topic under question that will both help the reader identify his relative strengths and weaknesses and fill any gaps in his knowledge. Useful references, for the most part drawn from readily available textbooks and journals, are provided.

The following general remarks should form the basis of your approach in the oral examination:

(1) Listen carefully to the question. The apprehensive candidate will frequently hear only a word or part of a question and answer accordingly, leaving the examiners with the impression that the specific question is being purposely avoided.

(2) Talk when you are allowed to do so. It is important to start answering quickly and avoid silences.

(3) Ensure that your opening response to a question is pertinent and incisive. Do not become embroiled in a lengthy preliminary outline on the subject and only deal with the more minor aspects after you have detailed the main points.

(4) Avoid errors of commission. While errors of omission will be frequently overlooked in oral examinations, errors of commission will be painfully obvious.

(5) Avoid using jargon or abbreviations. If you use technical terms they should be defined immediately as the examiner may not be familiar with their meaning and will be irritated.

Good Luck!

Dublin, 1988

P M
E G

Acknowledgements

We wish to acknowledge the helpful comments of Dr Martina Corry and Dr Frank O'Donoghue and to express our appreciation to Miss Finola O'Brien for her secretarial assistance.

PATRICK McKEON
EILISH GILVARRY

Contents

1
Questions

1 What are the features of psychogenic pain and how is it treated?

2 What is a 'normal' grief reaction?

3 What are pseudohallucinations?

4 How would you make a diagnosis of mania?

5 What forms of the cognitive dysfunction are encountered in depression?

6 Is a subjective feeling of depression ever a feature of mania?

7 Which neuroleptic would you choose in treating acute schizophrenia?

8 What are the clinical features of school refusal?

9 What are the features of transsexualism?

10 What use is made of the Weschsler Adult Intelligence Scales?

11 What haematological and metabolic disturbances, other than endocrine changes, are encountered in anorexia nervosa?

12 What are the clinical and pathological features of Creutzfeldt-Jacob disease?

13 How effective is the detection and treatment of the suicidal patient in general practice?

14 What are the multiaxial systems of classification in child psychiatry?

15 Outline the general cognitive techniques used in treating depressive illness.

16 What is the role of the psychogeriatric team?

17 What is subcortical dementia?

18 What electroencephalographic abnormalities would you expect to see in subjects with psychopathic personalities and what are their significance?

19 What are the causes of severe mental handicap?

20 Outline the characteristics of hallucinations.

21 What is the link between psychiatric disorder and deliberate self harm?

22 Do children show a bereavement reaction?

23 Define the term alexithymia.

24 How would you select patients for group psychotherapy?

25 What is cognitive therapy?

26 Which depot neuroleptic would you choose in maintenance therapy of schizophrenia?

27 Are there differences in the clinical presentaton of depression in the elderly?

28 What factors pertain to the use of tricyclic anti-depressants in nocturnal enuresis?

29 What are the features of the chronic amnesic syndrome and how is it distinguished from dementia?

30 What are the clinical features of Turner's syndrome?

31 What are the psychological consequences of cancer?

32 Is there an association between social class and mental handicap?

33 How is dopamine implicated in the pathogenesis of schizophrenia?

34 What is the significance of the Face-Hand test?

35 What constitutes a psychiatric emergency?

36 What are the clinical features of Kleinefelter's syndrome?

37 What is akathisia?

38 What effect does electroconvulsive therapy have on EEG recordings taken between treatments and when do the changes revert?

39 How would you manage the suicidal person?

40 What psychological approaches could you use in the management of dementia?

41 What laboratory findings would help identify the problem drinker?

42 What are the major disadvantages associated with barbiturate drugs in psychiatric practice?

43 In what conditions do hallucinations occur?

44 Do mentally handicapped children suffer from the same psychiatric disorders as those with normal intelligence?

45 What are first rank symptoms?

46 Is there an increased psychiatric morbidity after hysterectomy?

47 Are suicide and bereavement associated?

48 What are the clinical features of volatile substance abuse?

49 What is the masquerade syndrome?

50 What are the epidemiological aspects of parasuicide?

51 How would you manage a manic patient presenting as an emergency?

52 What are the range of functions of a liaison psychiatrist?

53 In what disorders might cognitive therapy be beneficial?

54 How would you diagnose schizophrenia in the mentally handicapped person?

55 How should late paraphrenia be managed and what is its outcome?

56 To what does the term 'dementia' refer?

57 Are there any contraindications to performing a lumbar puncture?

58 Is mental illness associated with an increased risk of suicide?

59 What is the outcome of school refusal?

60 What are the major treatment methods in a rehabilitation programme for schizophrenics?

61 What are cognitive distortions?

62 What physical complications do opiate addicts suffer from? What is the mortality rate?

63 What forms do pathological grief reactions take?

64 What prognostic factors have been identified in anorexia nervosa?

65 Outline the characteristics of the neuroleptic malignant syndrome?

66 List some of the psychological measures used in assessment of the mentally handicapped child.

67 What disorders would you consider in the differential diagnosis of schizophrenia?

68 What is the premenstrual syndrome? Is there a link with psychiatric disorders?

69 What clinically derived classifications of depression are you familiar with?

70 How would you manage the opiate addict?

71 What is the punch drunk syndrome?

72 What are the causes of Wernicke's encephalopathy?

73 What are aspects of management for sexual dysfunction?

74 What is the incidence of homosexuality?

75 What is the long term outcome of depression in the elderly and what are considered to be prognostic indicators?

76 What are tics and how are they treated?

77 What is the evidence for a genetic contribution in schizophrenia?

78 Is there an association between substance abuse and suicidal behaviour?

79 What medication might benefit the schizophrenic patient who appears resistant to neuroleptics?

80 What does the term 'curative factors' mean in group psychotherapy? List these factors.

81 What changes do psychiatric medications have on EEG recordings?

82 What clinically derived classifications of depression are you familiar with?

83 What is the association between psychiatric illness and bereavement?

84 Outline the behavioural approaches used in the treatment of sexual deviations.

85 What are the causes of increased psychiatric disorder in mentally handicapped children?

86 What are the clinical features of infantile autism

87 What methods are used in deliberate self harm?

88 Does high expressed emotion have a causal role in schizophrenia?

89 What theories of suicide did Durkheim propound?

90 How would you distinguish between psychogenic and organic amnesia?

91 What are the prevalence rates for neuroses and personality disorders in the elderly?

92 Are CAT scans of value in the management of dementia syndromes?

93 How would you assess the suicidal risk in a patient who has recently attempted suicide?

94 How useful are EEG recordings in psychiatry?

95 You suspect that a patient has neurosyphilis. What test would you do and how would you interpret the results?

96 What are the diagnostic criteria for anorexia nervosa?

97 Outline Piaget's stages of cognitive development.

98 What psychometric tests would help differentiate between depression and dementia?

99 What is the Hamilton Rating Scale?

100 How useful is a brain CAT scan to a psychiatrist?

101 How should the mental handicap team help the families of handicapped children?

102 What measures might help prevent mental handicap?

103 How would you manage a transsexual patient?

104 What types of hallucinations are seen in schizophrenia?

105 What are the clinical features of the opiate withdrawal syndrome?

106 What is morbid jealousy and with what is it associated?

107 What are mood congruent delusions?

108 You have been asked to assess a patient for behaviour modification, discuss in general terms how you would proceed.

109 Does parasuicide increase the risk of suicide?

110 What is dysmorphophobia?

111 With what sexual problems do male homosexuals present to a psychiatrist? How are they treated?

112 Outline the characteristics of the elderly alcoholic. What is the prevalence of alcoholism in the elderly population?

113 How would you manage a child with faecal soiling?

114 What is meant by the term 'expressed emotion'?

115 What are the clinical features of late paraphrenia?

116 You have been called to assess a patient who has recently taken an overdose. How would you proceed?

117 What are the characteristics of a transvestite?

118 What is retrograde amnesia and what is its significance?

119 What personality characteristics are associated with drug abuse?

120 Is there a genetic component to the development of alcoholism?

121 How common are the chronic psychiatric sequelae of head injury?

122 How would you decide whether a patient is sleeping or in a coma?

123 What factors are associated with repetition of parasuicide?

124 How would you treat depression in schizophrenia?

125 Is there a role for cognitive therapy in eating disorders?

126 What disorders would you consider in the differential diagnosis of autism and how are they distinguished?

127 What forms of psychiatric disorder follow amphetamine abuse?

128 Outline the language disorder of schizophrenia.

129 Does the patient with Klinefelter's syndrome show an increased psychiatric vulnerability?

130 What is institutionalism?

131 What are the main components of a social skills training programme?

132 What are the different concepts of schizo-affective disorder?

133 What is the post-concussional syndrome?

134 What is the prognosis for drug addiction and what features are of predictive value?

135 What social factors are associated with suicide?

136 What are the causes of depression in schizo-phrenia?

137 What factors are associated with repetition of parasuicide?

138 What are the methods used in suicide?

139 What kind of personality changes might you find in a patient with organic brain damage?

140 Outline the major sociological aspects of drug abuse.

141 How would you manage an alcohol withdrawal syndrome?

142 What is the psychodynamic view of manic behaviour?

143 What are flight of ideas? In what conditions do they occur?

144 Have depot neuroleptics any advantage over oral neuroleptics?

145 You have been asked to prepare a court report on a patient who has sustained a head injury. What should be the salient aspects of such a report?

146 What is the frequency of sexual problems in the general population?

147 Differentiate clinically between multi-infarct dementia and senile dementia.

148 What interventions are used in family management of schizophrenia?

149 How do patterns of friendship change through adolescence?

150 Is there an organic basis for aggressive behaviour?

151 Outline the characteristics of the exhibitionist.

152 What are the Research Diagnostic Criteria?

153 What are the main indications for the use of electroconvulsive therapy?

154 What are paranoid states?

155 What are the clinical features of bulimia nervosa?

156 What are the features of suicide in hospitalised psychiatric patients?

157 Define thought block.

158 How would you clinically assess a patient with suspected dementia?

159 What chromosomal abnormalities are associated with Down's syndrome?

160 What are the characteristics of those who physically abuse children?

161 What are the medical and psychiatric complications associated with chronic use of cannabis?

162 What are the features of the different clinical subtypes of bipolar manic-depressive illness?

163 Are cerebral tumours misdiagnosed in psychiatric practise? What are the common modes of presentation?

164 What is the recommended management of depersonalisation?

165 How common is depression in chronic schizophrenia?

166 How would you manage the enuretic child?

167 What laboratory and radiological investigations would you consider when investigating dementia?

168 How would you differentiate clinically between dementia and depressive pseudodementia?

169 What are psychomotor seizures and how do they manifest?

170 What are the main features of the frontal lobe syndrome?

171 How common is suicide in schizophrenia and are there predictive features?

172 Have social class factors been implicated in the aetiology of schizophrenia?

173 What is the Gilles de la Tourette syndrome and how is it treated?

174 How would you assess a patient who deliberately harms himself?

175 What is a neologism?

176 What is the DSM III and how does it differ from the DSM II?

177 Is there an 'epileptic personality'?

178 What are the clinical features of benzodiazepine withdrawal?

179 What is the relationship between recent life events and depression?

180 What types of faecal soiling are seen in children?

181 What is 'pseudodementia'? List its causes.

182 What are the causes of erectile dysfunction?

183 What uses has day hospital care for the elderly with dementia?

184 What is the relationship between epilepsy and psychosis?

185 How common is depression?

186 What are the manifestations of physical abuse in children?

187 What is an illusion?

188 What is the Guthrie test and how is it interpreted?

189 What is the suicide rate in England? Is it increasing?

190 What are the effects of cocaine?

191 What evidence is there to support a genetic contribution to the development of bipolar manic-depression?

192 Is cognitive impairment associated with Parkinson's syndrome?

193 What are the psychological manifestations of a diencephalic lesion?

194 What features of schizophrenia have prognostic significance?

195 What is meant by specific retardation? Outline its prevalence and clinical features.

196 What social support facilities are available for the elderly?

197 Describe the two-syndrome concept in schizophrenia.

198 What factors are involved in the development of antisocial behaviour?

199 How would you assess a man who is complaining of erectile dysfunction?

200 What is the outcome of anorexia nervosa?

201 Where are the electrodes usually applied for bilateral electroconvulsive therapy?

202 What factors determine the differences in a person's response to grief?

203 Describe the Eysenck Personality Inventory?

204 Is electroconvulsive therapy useful in schizophrenia?

205 How would you routinely assess a cognitive function?

206 What is cannabis?

207 What are passivity phenomena?

208 Do psychiatric disorders in adolescence remit?

209 What is the association between affective disorders and Parkinson's syndrome?

210 What causes tardive dyskinesia and how should it be treated?

211 What factors are associated with enuresis?

212 Describe the clinical features of multi-infract dementia.

213 With what psychodynamic explanations of depression are you familiar?

214 What is the importance of the domiciliary visit in the assessment of the elderly?

215 How would you interview and manage an acutely paranoid patient who presents as an emergency?

216 What is covert sensitisation and for what is it used?

217 What disorders would you consider in the differential diagnosis of stupor and what are their distinguishing features?

218 What psychiatric manifestations of General Paresis of the Insane are encountered in present day clinical practice.

219 What is dermatitis artefacta?

220 What complications are associated with electro-convulsive therapy?

221 What is the General Health Questionnaire and what use is made of it?

222 Are female alcoholics different from their male counterparts?

223 What are the characteristics of incest victims?

224 Describe the clinical features of anorexia nervosa?

225 What are the consequences for the victims of child sexual abuse?

226 What is insight?

227 What are the features of cannabis intoxication?

228 How would you manage a depressed stroke patient?

229 What are the usual wave patterns on the standard E.E.G. and how do they vary with age?

230 Outline the autonomic effects of the phenothiazines.

231 What are the differences between school refusal and school truancy?

232 Describe the clinical features of Alzheimer's disease.

233 What is the prevalence of dementia?

234 How would you treat alcoholic hallucinosis and what is its prognosis?

235 Who would benefit from social skills training?

236 Would you expect to see changes in an E.E.G. recording in a patient with a chronic subdural haematoma?

237 What psychiatric symptoms might you expect in cerebral systemic lupus erythematosus?

238 How would you treat a pathological grief reaction?

239 What is the Rorschach test, how is it interpreted and what is its present status in clinical practice?

240 What are the indications for unilateral ECT and where are the electrodes usually placed?

241 Outline the general principles for treating anorexia nervosa.

242 What behavioural methods are most effective in treating obsessional disorders?

243 Outline the side effects of the anticholinergic drugs.

244 How would you manage a patient with a suspected conversion symptom of recent onset?

245 What is the outcome of infantile autism?

246 What are the practical implications of drug prescribing in the elderly?

247 What factors are thought to contribute to the development of anorexia nervosa?

248 What routine do you follow for a pre-ECT work-up after a decision has been made to give the treatment?

249 What hormonal changes occur in anorexia nervosa?

250 What are the features of the Capgras syndrome and what is its aetiology?

251 What are the differences between early and late onset childhood psychoses?

252 Are psychiatric patients more likely to have vitamin B12 deficiency and what are the common psychiatric manifestations of such a deficiency?

253 How would you distinguish between a diagnosis of depressive disorder and anxiety neurosis when symptoms of both are present?

254 Who sniffs glue? How common is this form of substance abuse?

255 Define negativism. What disorders is it associated with?

256 How would you withdraw a patient from benzodiazepines?

257 Should anticholinergic drugs be routinely used with neuroleptic medication?

258 What is elective mutism? Describe its clinical features.

259　What drugs might help improve cerebral function in senile dementia?

260　What depressive features predict a favourable treatment response to ECT?

261　What do you mean by biofeedback? What are the indications for its use?

262　How common is anorexia nervosa? Are prevalence and incidence rates increasing?

263　What is Asperger's syndrome?

264　What are the current indications for psychosurgery?

265　What is the Ganser syndrome and how is it distinguished from Ganser symptoms?

266　Describe the clinical presentation of stupor. What are its causes?

267　Describe the foetal alcohol syndrome.

268　What is myxoedema madness and who first described it?

269　What is the basis for the use of the Dexamethasone Suppression Test in psychiatry and how useful is it?

270　What are the 'hallucinogenic drugs'? What effects do they produce?

271　What aetiological factors are implicated in the hyperkinetic syndrome?

272　What is meant by the term 'tolerance' with reference to therapeutics? How does it occur?

273　Outline the causes of mutism.

274　What is the relevance of the thyrotropin releasing hormone test in affective disorders?

275　Which of the porphyrias are relevant to psychiatry and how would you investigate a suspected case?

276　Define the terms flooding and implosion therapy. Outline the procedures.

277　What is acute dystonia?

278 How would you manage the child with school refusal?

279 Describe the pathology of Alzheimer's disease.

280 What commonly used drugs interact with the phenothiazines?

281 What is systematic desensitisation and how is it used to treat phobic disorders?

282 What are the psychiatric symptoms associated with hypoglycaemia?

283 What personality traits are associated with unipolar and bipolar affective disorders?

284 What are the characteristics of an emotionally deprived child?

285 How would you distinguish between perseveration and a verbal stereotypy?

286 Describe the features of the Othello syndrome?

287 What are the more common psychosurgical operations?

288 How would you manage the bulimic patient?

289 What is the relationship between adult psychiatric disorders and their childhood precursors?

290 What are the features of Munchausen's syndrome and how does it present?

291 What is the fragile-X syndrome?

292 Identify the features of the alcohol dependence syndrome.

293 Are the psychiatric manifestations of Cushing's disease the same as those associated with steroids administered for therapeutic purposes?

294 Outline the metabolic and endocrine effects of the phenothiazines.

295 What features best differentiate Pick's disease from Alzheimer's disease?

296 What is the punch drunk syndrome?

297 What is orgasmic conditioning?

298 Are there any mental symptoms associated with hypercalcaemia?

299 How would you manage a patient with lithium toxicity?

300 What are the clinical features of tardive dyskinesia and what disorders would you consider in its different diagnosis?

301 What pharmacokinetic factors influence the action of psychotropic drugs in the elderly?

302 How would you treat an acute grief reaction?

303 What is token economy?

304 How might a phaeochromocytoma present to a psychiatrist and what clinical features would help to support the diagnosis?

305 Describe the characteristics of delusions.

306 What is the prognosis for treated and untreated alcoholism?

307 Is there a role for drug prescribing in the management of sexual dysfunction?

308 How would you recognise the problem drinker?

309 What forms of mental disturbance occur in uraemia?

310 How would you manage an acutely disabling anxiety state?

311 How would you treat insomnia in the elderly?

312 What evidence is there to support the entity of 'endogenous depression' and can it be distinguished from other forms of depression?

313 Describe the alcohol withdrawal syndrome.

314 What is the basis for the belief of being possessed?

315 What complications are associated with psycho-surgery?

316 Do sociocultural factors influence the development of anorexia nervosa?

317 What patterns of psychiatric disorder are found in an adolescent population?

318 What are the clinical features of Down's syndrome?

319 What are the neurological and neuropsychiatric complications of alcoholism?

320 What range of psychiatric syndromes are associated with multiple sclerosis?

321 What is the differential diagnosis of memory impairment in a fifty-five year old man?

322 What are the demographic characteristics of childhood suicide?

323 What is spasmodic torticollis and how should it be treated?

324 How would you recognise the elderly alcoholic?

325 How prevalent is mental illness in non-Western cultures?

326 How does Wernicke encephalopathy present?

327 What are night terrors?

328 What are the clinical features of Korsakoff's syndrome?

329 Describe the features of phenylketonuria.

330 How useful are psychometric tests of cognitive function?

331 Outline the structural and neurochemical difference between Alzheimer's Type I and II.

332 What is Amok?

333 What is the rationale for prescribing disulfiram and what are its side-effects?

334 What is operant conditioning? Outline its uses.

335 What are the features of Briquet's syndrome?

336 Are there reversible dementias?

337 Describe the pathological changes in Wernicke-Korsakoff's syndrome.

338 How would you manage a patient with 'morbid jealousy'?

339 What is the significance of the Face-Hand test?

340 Can hysterical personality traits be distinguished from hysteria?

341 What is the nature of the association between depression and the menopause?

342 How would you assess the likelihood of recurrence of violent behaviour and make recommendation to a court?

343 You have been asked to speak to a patient with bipolar manic-depression of the risk of one of his children developing a mood disorder—what factual information would form the basis for your approach?

344 What is the relationship between mental illness and shoplifting?

345 What are considered to be the selection criteria for short-term psychotherapy?

346 Can monoamine oxidase inhibitors be safely prescribed along with other psychotropics?

347 What are the features of a lithium induced tremor and how should it be managed?

348 To what does the term 'masked depression' refer?

349 What factors contribute to the development of juvenile delinquency?

350 How would you assess and manage an instance of possible baby battering?

351 Does clomipramine have any advantage over other tricyclic antidepressants in the treatment of depression?

352 How effective is lithium in the treatment and prophylaxis of bipolar manic-depressive illness?

353 What are phobias and how are they classified?

354 What is transactional analysis and what is its theoretical basis?

355 What is the relationship, if any, between obsessive compulsive neurosis and schizophrenia?

356 What is the legal concept of infanticide?

357 What factors are thought to contribute to the formation of phobias?

358 How would you identify resistance in analytical psychotherapy?

359 How would you define obsessive-compulsive neurosis?

360 What is the prognosis for the different phobic disorders?

361 What are the main traits of schizoid personality?

362 What is hypochondriasis?

363 What features characterise the sociopathic personality?

364 Is stress a factor in the genesis of obsessive compulsive neurosis?

365 What is meant by the term 'narcissistic reaction' and why do patients who have such reactions pose a problem in psychotherapy?

366 Is mental illness more prevalent among prisoners and what are the more commonly occurring psychiatric disorders in mentally abnormal offenders?

367 Who can discharge a patient who has been compulsorily admitted to hospital in England?

368 How should a psychopathic person who has received a criminal conviction be managed?

369 When is a plea of diminished responsibility used and what is its significance?

370 What are the main features of obsessional personality?

371 What is the relationship between the 47 XYY syndrome and criminal behaviour?

372 What is 'la belle indifference'?

373 You have been asked by the relatives of an elderly intermittently confused man whether he is mentally fit to make a will. How would you assess his fitness?

374 What are considered to be the contraindications for brief psychotherapy?

375 What legal procedures are available to the person who through illness is not able to manage his affairs?

376 What is the incidence of post-natal depression and how likely is it to recur? What aetiological factors are associated with the different syndromes?

377 How should individual psychotherapy be terminated?

378 What are the recommended laboratory and clinical assessments for patients taking lithium prophylactically?

379 What is the present status of plasma tricyclic antidepressant estimations in clinical practice?

380 How would you make a diagnosis of anxiety neurosis?

381 What side effects are associated with serum lithium levels which are within the therapeutic range?

382 What are the main indications for prescribing monoamine oxidase inhibitors?

383 What would you consider for the differential diagnosis in the case of a fifty year old man who presents for the first time with syptoms of acute anxiety?

384 What are the difficulties in diagnosing depression in general practice?

385 You are about to prescribe tricyclic antidepressants, what advice would you give the patient about the medication and how would you initiate treatment?

386 What are the indications and techniques for supportive psychotherapy?

387 What personal qualities in the therapist are considered to be necessary for effective psychotherapy?

388 You suspect that a patient with limb paralysis has a hysterical conversion syndrome—how would you clarify the diagnosis?

389 Do murderers have a typical profile?

390 What are the more common side effects associated with trimipramine?

391 Can tricyclic antidepressants be prescribed during pregnancy?

392 What is countertransference and how should it be managed?

393 What are the psychological reactions to rape?

394 An obstetrician has asked you about the management of lithium during pregnancy—what advice would you give?

395 What serum lithium concentration is therapeutically desirable?

396 A patient with bipolar manic-depression who is taking lithium on a prophylactic basis and is currently in remission has asked about the possibility of terminating treatment—what would you advise?

397 How is acting out in psychotherapy best managed?

398 How would you treat an acutely manic patient?

399 How would you manage a person who has been charged with indecent exposure?

2
Answers

1 Pain occurring in the absence of an adequate physical explanation and in the presence of causative psychological factors is usually referred to as psychogenic pain. The diagnosis is usually made after investigation and exclusion of organic pathology. The patient is commonly a middle aged female who complains of chronic and continuous pain throughout the day that may prevent her getting off to sleep, but does not awaken her. The main sites of pain are the head, neck, face, lower back and abdomen and the sensations are often described as occurring in areas which are inconsistent with anatomical nerve distribution. Insight into the role of psychological factors is often restricted. The course is variable and is dependent on reinforcement factors such as litigation process, current social stresses and secondary gains. The pain responds better to psychotropics than analgesic medication. If pain is a feature of psychiatric illness, particularly depression, antidepressants should be prescribed. Pain clinics run by a psychiatrist, physician and anaesthetist have been established and medication, psychotherapy and behavioural techniques are commonly used.

Pilowsky I 1983 Chronic pain: The role of the psychiatrist. In: Russell G, Hersov L (eds) The neuroses and personality disorders. Handbook of Psychiatry 4. Cambridge University Press, Cambridge

2 Grief reactions typically proceed through a series of stages. The immediate reaction consists of a period of numbness lasting from hours to days which is sometimes preceded by a brief period of distress, tearfulness and occasionally panic attacks. After 5 to 7 days a sharp increase in affective symptoms occur, often with intense pining for the deceased. Other symptoms include preoccupation with thoughts of the deceased, anxiety, restlessness, futility feelings, anorexia and loss of interest in personal appearance. Perceptual

25

disturbances such as illusions, misidentifications, pseudohallucinations and a sense of the presence of the deceased may occur. Restlessness may be associated with searching behaviour and clinging to the deceased's possessions. Bereaved persons are often angry, preoccupied with self-blame or project the blame on to others and they frequently idealise the dead person. There are wide variations between individuals in the time course of events but the intensity of the distress generally diminishes over weeks and depressive symptoms last for many months, until re-adjustment occurs. The whole process is considered to take six months but anniversaries are often a time of renewed grieving.

Parkes C 1972 Bereavement. Studies of grief in adult life. Penguin, London

3   Jaspers described pseudohallucinations as a form of imagery rather than as perceptions. They are subjective, have no concrete validity and are observed within the person's mind and not in outer objective space, while hallucinations are perceived as occurring in outer objective space. Pseudohallucinations are not under voluntary control but the patient generally realises that they are occurring in his mind. A person with a pseudo-hallucination of hearing a voice saying 'pull yourself together' would acknowledge that this voice was an inner voice, occurring in subjective space and would usually describe it as the voice of conscience. Pseudohallucinations differ from mental images in that they are not under voluntary control. Mental images are also inconstant, not clearly delineated and are incomplete. Pseudohallucinations may occur in all forms of psychotic disturbance, in disturbed states of consciousness and in normal individuals.

Mullen P E 1986 The mental state and states of mind. In: Hill P, Murray R, Thorley A (eds) Essentials of Postgraduate Psychiatry, 2nd edn. Grune and Stratton, London

4   Increased energy, over-talkativeness, flight of ideas, distractability, uninhibited behaviour and initial insomnia with early morning wakening are the main features of mania or hypomania. Initially the patient may be humorous and euphoric, but can quickly become irritable and angry when thwarted. For some, particularly those who are having hypomanic moods while on lithium, the

mood has a definite dysphoric quality in that the patient will complain of irritability, tension, mental restlessness and depression while exhibiting behavioural hyperactivity. The grandiose plans and a tendency to perceive only the positive aspects of any situation underlies the impaired judgement of mania. The grandiose over-valued ideas frequently become delusional and their content usually centres on the political, financial, sexual or religious domain. While it is generally accepted that manic patients have delusions and hallucinations which are affectively based, they also can have schizophreniform features: a survey of a large series of studies reported that 20–50% of manic patients experience delusions of persecution, catatonic symptoms or Schneiderian first rank symptoms. In the early stage of hypomania the patient is usually unaware of the change in mood and on occasions family members may not be concerned about the elation when it is occurring after a prolonged bout of depression. So, in order not to overlook a diagnosis of hypomania or mania the patient's premorbid personality must be enquired about in detail.

Taylor S, Abrams R 1973 The phenomenology of mania: A new look at some old patients. Archives of General Psychiatry 29: 520–522

Tyrer S, Shopsin B 1982 Symptoms and assessment of mania. In: Paykel E S (ed) Handbook of Affective Disorders. Churchill Livingstone, Edinburgh

5 Depressed patients typically demonstrate the following: automatic intrusive thoughts that are irrational and maladaptive, cognitive distortions which bias the patient's view of reality and primary assumptions which add to the patient's tendency to develop depression. Automatic intrusive thoughts are rapidly occurring thoughts and images that accompany or immediately precede the individual's reaction to an internally or externally occurring event. In depressed patients these thoughts are irrational, maladaptive and self-defeating and examples of these are: 'they are all laughing at me', 'failed again', 'no one cares'. Cognitive distortions or processing errors are ways of thinking that bias the patient's view of reality. Common examples include arbitary inference, over-generalisation, selective abstraction, dichotomous thinking and magnification. Primary assumptions involve inflexible rules related to self-

evaluation or to relationships with others, for example: 'my value as a person depends on the respect others show me', 'I must make my life worthwhile everyday or else I am worthless'. Beck has summarised the cognitive disorder resulting from these errors of thinking as a cognitive triad, the three components being a negative view of one's self, a negative interpretation of current experience and a negative view of the future.

Beck A T 1963 Thinking and depression I. Idiosyncratic content and cognitive distortions. Archives of General Psychiatry 9: 324–333
Beck A T 1964 Thinking and depression II. Theory and therapy. Archives of General Psychiatry 10: 561–571

6   A transient feeling of depression is reported to occur in some 70% of manic patients. For a minority this may be the main presenting complaint and the predominant symptom during the manic phase. However, features of behavioural hyperactivity such as pressure of speech, flight of ideas and motor hyperactivity will distinguish the manic state from the hypoactivity of the depressive phase.

A dysphoric mood is more commonly encountered in manic patients who have inadequate serum lithium concentrations. The heightened sense of empathy associated with mania may also produce shortlived episodes of tearfulness and sadness.

Kukopulos A, Reginaldi D 1980 Recurrences of manic-depressive episodes during lithium treatment. In: Johnson F N (ed) Handbook of Lithium Therapy M T P Press, Lancaster
Winokur G, Clayton P, Reich P 1969 In: Manic-Depressive Illness. C V Mosby, St Louis

7   There is a bewildering choice of drugs available— the phenothiazines, butyrophenones, diphenyl-butylpiperidines, indole derivatives, thiozanthenes and the benzamide derivatives. The choice of drug is governed mainly by the desirability of sedation, the pattern of side-effects tolerated by the individual patient and the frequency of dosage required. Most of the neuroleptics show some anticholinergic, anti-adrenergic, extrapyramidal and sedative properties. Chlorpromazine, with its marked sedative properties, may be useful in the acutely psychotic patient. However, its sedative

effects and extrapyramidal effects may be a draw-back. If over-sedation is a problem one of the piperazine compounds such as trifluoperazine may be useful. This drug is reported to have a 'stimulating' effect, but is accompanied by an increase in extrapyramidal effects. In contrast thioridazine has less extrapyramidal effects but is more likely to cause hypotension and ejaculatory failure. Pimozide and fluspirilene have a low incidence of extrapyramidal effects and are claimed to be of special value in inert and apathetic schizophrenics. They may be useful if compliance is a problem. Benzamides, for example the sulpirides, are said to have little sedative action. The butyrophenones have much the same action as the phenothiazines but with a greater tendency to produce extrapyramidal side-effects and akathisia. Neither the thioxanthenes nor butyrophenones have any advantage over the phenothiazines and research has failed to show any significant differences in overall efficacy between one neuroleptic phenothiazine and another. However, while there seems little difference in efficacy, individual variation in response may be marked. Differences in response may be mediated more by individual differences among patients than by differences between the drugs.

Johnstone E 1985 Acute schizophrenia. British Journal of Hospital Medicine 34(4): 198–201

McClelland H 1986 Treatment in schizophrenia: Overview. In: Kerr A, Snaith P (eds) Contemporary Issues in Schizophrenia. Gaskell Psychiatry Series

8 The problem starts with vague complaints about school or reluctance to attend, progressing to total refusal to go to school despite parental and school pressure. The child may simply refuse to go to school, refuse to remain at school or may develop overt panic just before school time. In some instances the child complains of many somatic problems such as anorexia, nausea, vomiting, syncope, abdominal pain, headache and vague malaise. These complaints occur in the morning before school and subside when the child is allowed to stay at home. Obsessional symptoms sometimes occur. There may be marked depressive features and suicidal behaviour may follow. The sex ratio is equal and the most common age at presentation is eleven years. The child stays at home with the parents' knowledge and they are

generally very concerned over the non-attendance. School refusal is typically manifested in children who are timid, shy and dependent and they come from average sized families. Their academic achievements are normal or superior and their behaviour at school is exemplary. An acute onset is usually seen in young children whereas in older children and adolescence there is usually a more insidious onset. Precipitating factors are common such as change of school or teacher, bereavement or departure of a friend. The older child gradually withdraws from his peer group, clings to the mother and ceases to go out. Closer observation may reveal behavioural problems, depression or, rarely, a psychotic illness. Among younger children the fear is more of separation from an attachment figure. Mothers tend to be over protective and approximately 25% of the mother of school refusers suffer from a psychiatric disorder, more often of an affective nature.

Berg I 1984 School refusal. British Journal Hospital Medicine 31 (1): 59–63
Hersov L 1985 School refusal. In: Rutter M, Hersov L (eds) Child and Adolescent Psychiatry, 2nd edn. Blackwell, London

9   This is a psychosexual condition in which a member of either sex has an over-riding compulsion to live in the gender role appropriate to a person of the opposite biological sex. This paradoxical gender identity is usually permanent and unchangeable and typically manifests before puberty. Generally the transsexual shows great distaste for his genitalia and secondary sex characteristics, shows little interest in sexual activity but is attracted to others of the same anatomical sex, while insisting that he is not homosexual. The behaviour and dress of the opposite sex is adopted, but in cross dressing no sexual arousal is experienced. They usually pursue sex re-assignment with fanatical fervour. Transsexuals generally have poor work records, despite average ability obtain poor qualifications, are more often of lower socio-economic group and have a high rate of psychiatric disturbance mainly of the neurotic and personality disordered categories. Males predominate in the ratio of 3 or 4:1. Hoenig and Kenna, reporting on the sexual orientation of transsexuals, claimed that nearly 10% were fetishistic, 40% homosexual and nearly 80% were

fetishistic transvestites before the full elaboration of their transsexualism. They found that only homosexuality persisted after the development of the syndrome.

Hoenig J, Kenna J C 1974(a) The nosological position of transsexualism. Archives of Sexual Behaviour 3: 273–287
Hoenig J, Kenna J C 1974(b) The prevalence of transsexualism in England and Wales. British Journal of Psychiatry 124: 181–190
Hoenig J 1982 Transsexualism In: Granville-Grossman K (ed) Recent Advances in Clinical Psychiatry. Churchill Livingstone, Edinburgh

10 This is an extensively standardised instrument for measuring intelligence and has the additional benefit of providing separate scores for verbal and performance abilities. It is also useful in detecting brain damage as changes from premorbid IQ can be assessed. A significantly higher verbal than performance score is indicative of brain damage as performance abilities are more susceptible to change. Lesions of the dominant cerebral hemisphere will effect comprehension, arithmetic and vocabulary subtests of the verbal scale, while leaving performance scores intact. However, significant discrepancies can occur in some normal subjects and in those with functional disorders. The WAIS has deterioration indices which help to assess brain damage. They contrast how the subject fares on subtests which are relatively impervious to change, that is the Information, Vocabulary, Object Assembly and Picture Completion subtests with those which deteriorate with brain damage: Digit Span, Similarities, Digit Symbol and Block Design. While these indices tend to correlate with the degree of diffuse brain damage, they have been criticied for their unreliability in distinguishing organic cases from functional disorders. However, the WAIS subtests are useful for detecting brain damage and they should be interpreted in conjunction with other clinical and psychological test data.

Cutting J, McClelland R 1986 Psychiatric manifestations of organic illness. In: Hill P, Murray R Thorley A (eds) Essentials of Postgraduate Psychiatry 2nd edn. Grune and Stratton London
Savage R D 1974 Intellectual assessment. In: Mittler P (ed) The Psychological Assessment of Mental and Physical Handicaps. Tavistock, London

11 Leucopenia, relative lymphocytosis and hypocellularity in the bone marrow are not unusual occurrences. Haemoglobin and sedimentation rate are usually normal but a mild iron and folic deficiency anaemia may occur. Plasma fibrinogen levels may be low with high plasminogen activator levels. The distorted diet is likely to lead to carotenaemia and high blood levels of cholesterol and urea from disproportionately high intakes of vegetables, cheese and protein respectively. Electrolytes are usually normal, but in patients who frequently vomit or abuse purgatives there may be a hypokalaemic alkalosis. Low glucose levels, abnormal glucose tolerance test and a raised insulin level are also common.

Fairburn C 1988 Eating disorders. In: Kendell R E, Zealley A K (eds) Companion to Psychiatric Studies, 4th edn. Churchill Livingstone, Edinburgh

12 This is a dementing illness with a sudden onset, which follows a rapid subsequent course and affects males and females equally. Clinically a psychiatric disorder may be suspected initially as anxiety, insomnia, depression, hypomanic behaviour or psychotic features may be the presenting symptoms. However, neurological features and intellectual impairment quickly ensue. The progressive intellectual deterioration evolves with great rapidity alongside the variable neurological features. These neurological features may include spasticity of limbs, myoclonic jerks and athethoid movements, extrapyramidal rigidity, cerebellar ataxia and lower motor neurone signs. Other features include dysarthria, cortical blindness and signs of parietal lobe involvement. Pathologically the essential features consist of neuronal degeneration, marked proliferation of astrocytes and frequently a characteristic spongy appearance of the grey matter. There is no definitive treatment for this dementia. A family history is rare and the disease almost always appears sporadically. However, rare cases have been reported with a familial pattern and a presumed genetic basis. It is thought that a transmissable agent similar to scarpie may account for some cases.

Bond M R, Kennedy R 1988 Organic disorders. In: Kendell R E, Zealley A K (eds) Companion to Psychiatric Studies, 4th edn. Churchill Livingstone, Edinburgh
Brain's Textbook of the Nervous System 8th edn, revised. 1977. J Walton, Oxford

13 Evidence from surveys of suicide victims who had been in contact with their family doctor before the event would suggest that the assessment and treatment of the suicidal patient is inadequate. Barraclough in 1974 reported that some two-thirds of suicide victims had seen their doctor a month before and 40% a week before their death. Over three-quarters were prescribed psychotropic drugs, but only one-third received an adequate course of antidepressant medication. Other studies have supported these findings. However, there is little information available on those who are successfully treated by the family practitioner. It is still not established whether therapeutic intervention has had an impact on suicide rates. Some, such as Brown (1979), claim that the fall in suicide rates are attributable to the reduced toxicity of domestic gas, the reduced lethality of prescribed drugs and improved treatment for self-poisoning. Barraclough, on the other hand, suggests that improved knowledge of the treatment of psychiatric illness has contributed to the fall in rates.

Brown J H 1979 Suicide in Britain. Archives of General Psychiatry 36: 1119–1124
Roy A 1982 Risk factors for suicide in psychiatric patients. Archives of General Psychiatry 39: 1089–1095

14 The two current and most widely used systems are the 9th edition of the International Classification of Diseases (ICD 9) and the 3rd Diagnostic and Statistical Manual (DSM III) of the American Psychiatric Association. They are both characterised by five diagnostic axes. The rationale for this system is that psychiatric diagnoses frequently involve several elements. The five axes of ICD 9 involve the following: clinical psychiatric syndrome, for example emotional disorder, specific delays in development such as speech delay or specific reading retardation, intellectual level, medical conditions such as eczema or diabetes and abnormal psychological conditions, for example family discord. The axes in DSM III are similar, though mental retardation is included in the psychiatric syndrome axis. The other main difference between the two systems is that ICD 9 uses a descriptive glossary for terms, while DSM III has introduced operationally defined diagnostic criteria.

American Psychiatric Association 1980 Diagnostic and statistical manual of mental disorder 3rd edn.

American Psychiatric Association, Washington, DC
World Health Organisation 1978 International
   Classification of Diseases 9th edn, revised. World
   Health Organisation, Geneva

15 Cognitive restructuring is the central component
of this therapy and consists of identifying the
maladaptive cognitions and substituting more
appropriate ways of thinking and behaving.
Behavioural components to therapy may include
problem solving skills, graded task assignments
and graduated activities to improve the apathy of
depressed patients. The initial stage in cognitive
re-structuring consists of eliciting the automatic
thoughts by keeping written records of moods and
thinking in everyday life and by describing
thoughts experienced during the interview. The
patient is asked to distance himself from the event
and examine systematically with the therapist the
evidence on which his subjective appraisal was
made. After challenging the assumptions, the
patient generates alternative ideas which are then
examined. Between sessions the patient closely
monitors and records his automatic thoughts and
task assignments. Reality testing is achieved
through role rehearsal and graded task assignments. During sessions the patient tries out new
ways of behaving and his performance on these
tasks is evaluated at the next session. The overall
programme is tightly organised and should be
managed in a moderately directive manner.

Beck A T, Rush A J, Shaw B F, Emery G 1979
   Cognitive therapy of depression. Wiley, New York
Gelder M 1985 Cognitive therapy. In: Granville-
   Grossman K (ed) Recent Advances in Clinical
   Psychiatry 5. Churchill Livingstone, Edinburgh

16 The team should offer common ground for all
disciplines to meet and discuss their clinical problems and responsibilities, to plan treatment
programmes and to contribute their individual
expertise to these programmes. Patients are
assessed by one or more member of the team in
domiciliary or hospital based settings. The team
should liaise with other hospital teams, community,
social and general practice services and voluntary
bodies. Support and advice should be available for
the families of elderly patients. Meetings are
conducted on a regular basis to discuss management of patients, standards of clinical practise,
problems and new ideas. The team should have

educative value for students, many medical and paramedical disciplines and the general public. Research, both clinical and operational, should be conducted by the team. Members include the psychogeriatric consultant, social workers, community psychiatric nurses and other hospital based nurses, psychologist, occupational therapist and physiotherapist.

Pitt B (ed) 1982 Psychogeriatrics: an introduction to the psychiatry of old age, 2nd edn. Churchill Livingstone, Edinburgh

17 This term describes the dementia that is seen in neurological disorders in which the primary degeneration involves subcortical structures such as the basal ganglia and brain stem. Albert and his colleagues outlined the concept of subcortical dementia in patients with supranuclear palsy. The concept has been enlarged to include the dementias associated with Parkinson's disease, Huntington's chorea, Wilson's disease, traumatic injuries, disseminated sclerosis, spinocerebellar degeneration and idiopathic calcification of the basal ganglia. The prominent clinical features include progressive intellectual impairment with forgetfulness and slowing of mental processes, personality and affective changes including apathy and depression. Unlike the cortical dementias, they do not have language and perceptual dysfunctions. While it is suggested that there is a clear division between cortical and subcortical dementias, as evidenced by the clinical presentation, anatomical involvement and neurochemical changes, a strict division seems difficult to accept as all dementias must affect widespread areas of the brain both cortical and subcortical.

Albert M L, Feldman R G, Willis A L 1974 The subcortical dementias of progressive supranuclear palsy. Journal of Neurology, Neurosurgery and Psychiatry 37: 121–130
Huber S, Paulson G 1985 The concept of subcortical dementia. American Journal of Psychiatry 142: 1312–1317

18 A higher frequency of bilateral rhythmic theta activity in central and temporal regions is the main feature, along with alpha variants and episodic posterior temporal slow wave activity. Focal abnormalities in the posterior temporal lobes, often bilateral, are also frequently found.

The majority of these EEG changes reflect brain immaturity and they would be considered normal in a younger age group. Both the antisocial behaviour and brain wave pattern improve with time.

Lishman W A 1978 Clinical assessment. In: Organic Psychiatry. Blackwell, Oxford

19 An aetiological factor is identifiable in 85% of those with severe subnormality. Down's syndrome is the most common cause with the fragile X syndrome second in frequency. Other inherited defects include tuberous sclerosis, phenylketonuria and other inborn errors of metabolism, X-linked disorders such as Hunter's syndrome, Lesch-Nyhan syndrome and some sex chromosome disorders. There are a multitude of external factors which may damage the brain or interfere with its development. Intrauterine infections such as rubella, cytomegalovirus or syphilis may cause severe handicap. Perinatal factors include prematurity, trauma, multiple births, anoxia, delayed labour and low birth weight. Postnatal factors include infections such as meningitis and encephalitis, metabolic abnormalities and status epilepticus. Accidents are responsible for increasing numbers and non-accidental injury account for 2–4% of children in subnormality hospitals.

Heaton-Ward W A, Wiley Y 1984 Mental Handicap. Wright, Bristol

20 They are false perceptions, perceived as occurring in objective space and are not sensory distortions or misinterpretations. They are experienced alongside normal perceptions and are not under voluntary control. They are perceived as having the qualities of real perceptions in that they are whole and vivid. Hallucinations differ from perceptions in that they come from 'within' even though the patient perceives them in objective space. They can affect all sensory modalities. Auditory hallucinations may vary in clarity and vary from buzzing sounds to a full running commentary. Schneider claims that specific types of auditory hallucinations are diagnostic of schizophrenia. Visual hallucinations may be elementary in the form of flashes of light, partly organised or completely organised as visions of people or objects. All visual hallucinations are particularly indicative of organic states. Hallucinations of smell, taste, touch, pains and deep sensation,

vestibular sensations and the hallucination of a presence may occur. Other special varieties of hallucination include functional hallucinations in which a stimulus which causes a hallucination is experienced as well as the hallucination; reflex hallucination in which a stimulus in one sensory field produces a hallucination in another; and extracampine hallucinations where the subject has a hallucination which is outside the limits of the sensory field.

Hamilton M 1984 (ed) Fish's clinical psychopathology, 3rd edn. Wright, Bristol

21 Most parasuicides have a recognisable form of psychiatric disorder and minor reactive depressive illnesses, in the face of situational upset, are the most common. A depressive syndrome is diagnosed in 35–79% but its severity is not related to the seriousness of the attempt. Attempters are often very impulsive, with personality disorders and social problems, but no specific personality disorder is implicated. Some 12% of parasuicides show evidence of a major psychiatric disorder, this usually being depressive or organic in type. Chronic problem drinking is a major feature of this population and it is part of the lifestyle of about 24% of men and 7% of women. Organic illness, epilepsy and mental retardation are also encountered more frequently than expected.

Kreitman N 1988 Suicide and parasuicide. In: Kendell R E, Zealley A K (eds) Companion to Psychiatric Studies, 4th edn. Churchill Livingstone, Edinburgh
Morgan H G 1982 Deliberate self-harm. In: Granville-Grossman K (ed) Recent Advances in Clinical Psychiatry 4. Churchill Livingstone, Edinburgh

22 Most children show a 'grieving' or depressive syndrome following the death of a parent that is normally short term and self-limiting but in some children abnormal patterns of behaviour may persist. Some children do not appear to grieve openly at all. The grief in children is characterised by sadness, crying, irritability, sleep disturbance, nightmares, general decrease in interests and poor school performance, sometimes culminating in early school drop out. This pattern seems to be universal in bereaved children but is particularly evident in older girls. Other symptoms include temper tantrums, uncontrollable aggression, conduct disorders and enuresis. Most of the

symptoms improve considerably within one year. There is some evidence that more severe depressive reactions occur in adolescent boys who have lost their fathers. The short-term nature of this grief pattern seems to depend on how the child's needs are met and how caring adults respond to them.

Van Eedeewegh M M, Bieri M, Parilla R H, Clayton P S 1982 The bereaved child. British Journal of Psychiatry 140: 23–29

Van Eedewegh M M, Clayton P S, Van Eedewegh P 1985 The bereaved child: Variables influencing early psychopathology. British Journal of Psychiatry 147: 188–194

23 This term coined by Sifneos, refers to a cognitive-affective disturbance that affects the way individuals experience and express their emotions and was first described as a feature of psychosomatic disorders. The essential features consist of a difficulty in identifying feelings, in distinguishing between feelings and body sensations, an inability to describe emotions to other people, an impoverished fantasy life and a preference for focusing on external events rather than inner experiences. The features are typically accompanied by a stiff and wooden facial appearance. Alexithymia is not confined to those with psychosomatic disorders and many with such disorders do not exhibit these behavioural characteristics. In general a supportive psychotherapeutic approach seems to be of some benefit.

Lesser I M 1981 A review of the Alexithymia concept. Psychosomatic Medicine 43: 531–543

Nemiah J C, Freyberger R, Sifneos P C 1976 Alexithymia: A view of the psychosomatic process. In: Hill O (ed) Modern Trends in Psychosomatic Medicine 3rd edn. Butterworth, London

24 Selection criteria vary widely depending on the structure, procedure and goals of group psychotherapy. As far as supportive and milieu groups are concerned such as in-patients and hostel groups, it is important to include all patients apart from those who are grossly disturbed. For therapy groups with specialised goals, patient selection is relatively uncomplicated: the admission criteria being simply the presence of the particular problems, for example, obesity, alcoholism, anorexia nervosa or a gambling problem. For dynamic psychotherapy the emphasis in selection criteria

is on exclusion of those patients who are unsuitable. Brain damaged, sociopathic, acutely psychotic, paranoid, narcissistic, actively suicidal and patients addicted to drugs or alcohol may either not benefit from the therapy or may be disruptive to other members. While there is an argument for having a mix of different personality types and problems so that the group interactions simulate real life situations, there is also a case for having patients who share common characteristics so that identifications can more easily be made. The best compromise is that the group members should have relatively similar degrees of maturity and comparable levels of intelligence. Social class, marital status, sex and occupation are of less importance and some admixture is advantageous in order to get a variety of opinions and reactions.

Yalom I 1975 (ed) The theory and practice of group therapy 2nd edn. Basic Books, New York.

25 It is a group of psychological treatments aimed at changing maladaptive cognitions. It derives from the ideas of Meichenbaum and Beck and has similarities to the rational emotive therapy introduced by Ellis. The main assumptions of cognitive therapy are that mood changes are caused by erroneous thought processes and that these distorted thinking patterns can be identified and modified by various verbal and behavioural techniques. The patient is trained to identify and record his automatic thoughts, to generate alternative and more adaptive thoughts and to test out alternative ways of thinking and behaving. A wide variety of techniques are used, such as explanation, challenging of assumptions, role rehearsal and modelling, homework assignments and problem solving techniques. Treatment is highly structured and moderately directive and is of relatively short duration.

MacKay D 1982 Cognitive behaviour therapy. British Journal of Hospital Medicine 27: 242–243

26 There are six depot preparations available: flupenthixol enanthate, clopenthixol decanoate, fluspirilene, haloperidol, fluphenazine enanthate and fluphenazine decanoate. These depot preparations have similar efficacy and toxicity. Their therapeutic and unwanted side-effects are broadly similar to their oral forms. Flupenthixol enanthate is claimed to have a specific antidepressant effect and it might be more useful in inert and apathetic

patients. Fluphenazine and clopenthixol have sedative properties and should be used in the aggressive patient. Haloperidol in depot form may be useful if there is any mood elevation. Fluspirilene has no sedative properties but needs to be administered weekly. Any difference in these depot preparations seems to centre on their relative sedative properties and their effect on mood.

Johnson D A W 1982 The long acting depot neuroleptics. In: Granville-Grossman K (ed) Recent Advances in Clinical Psychiatry No 4. Churchill Livingstone, Edinburgh

Murray R 1986 Schizophrenia. In: Hill P, Murray R, Thorley A (eds) Essentials of Postgraduate Psychiatry 2nd edn. Grune and Stratton, London

27 It is generally thought that, as depressives get older, their symptomatology is more often characterised by agitation rather than retardation and by self-reproach, anxiety and hypochondriacal ideas. Research findings show that there is no clinical picture peculiar to old age depression, though hypochondriacal symptoms are found significantly more often. Post described seven subtypes of depression; the 'organic' depression occurs where the affective symptoms are associated with dementia and depressive pseudodementia where the perplexity and apparent lack of awareness of surroundings gives the appearance of dementia. Other subtypes include the agitated reactive, neurotic, senile melancholia and masked varieties. In masked depression the patient's complaints are usually hypochondriacal. They may show biological features of depression such as weight loss, anorexia, sleep disturbance and deterioration in functional ability without mood change. The value of these subtypes lies in their description of clinical pictures rather than any sharp nosological distinctions. In most patients the diagnosis is not difficult and is made on the basis of a typical history, appearance, behaviour and thought content. Diagnostic difficulties may arise in differentiating depression from a dementing process and from schizophrenia or where there are no obvious depressive symptoms as in so called masked depression.

Jacoby R, Bergmann K 1986 In: Hill P, Murray R, Thorley A (eds) The psychiatry of old age 2nd edn. Grune and Stratton London

Levy R, Post F 1982 The psychiatry of late life. Blackwell, Oxford

28 A wide variety of drugs have been used in the treatment of enuresis but only the tricyclic antidepressants continue to have a significant role. The mechanism of the antidiuretic effect is unknown and it might be due to an antidepressant, anticholinergic, or an anxiolytic action or be related to an effect on brain activity during sleep. Imipramine will reduce wetting frequency in about 85% of children and will suppress it completely in about 30%. The clinical effect ceases in a substantial proportion who are still receiving medication. Relapse after withdrawal may be immediate or delayed but nearly all children will have returned to their usual wetting frequency three months after stopping the treatment. As their long term efficacy is in doubt, their therapeutic role is uncertain. However, because of the simplicity of their use and the rapidity of their effect, tricyclic antidepressants may be used on a short term basis to overcome an embarrassing situation or to temporarily reduce stresses within the family until behavioural techniques have been implemented. Side effects include dry mouth, blurring of vision, weight gain, convulsions and tremor and with larger doses ataxia, confusion and cardiac irregularities may occur. Standard dose regimes cannot be relied on and an individual treatment schedule has to be evolved for each child.

Blackwell B, Curran J 1973 The psychopharmacology of nocturnal enuresis. In: Kolvin I, MacKeith R, Meadow S (eds) Bladder Control and Enuresis. Clinics in Developmental medicine 48–49. Simp/Heinemann, London

29 The chronic amnesic syndrome refers to a disorder of memory particularly for recent events. In its pure form it is due to discrete lesions of the hippocampal lobes and a common example of this is Korsakoff's psychosis. It is distinguished from dementia by the absence of global deterioration of intellect.

Bond M R, Kennedy R I 1988 Organic disorders. In: Kendell R E, Zealley A K (eds) Companion to Psychiatric Studies, 4th edn. Churchill Livingstone, Edinburgh
Lishman W A 1978 Cardinal psychological features of cerebral disorder. In: Organic Psychiatry. Blackwell, Oxford

30 Patients with this syndrome have a 45 X chromosome constitution and they can be recognised at birth by the characteristic oedema of the hands and feet and loose skin fold around the neck. Clinical manifestations include webbing of the neck, prominent ears, broad chest with apparent wide spaced nipples, cubitus valgus and a stature which is always below the third percentile. Sexual maturation fails to occur at puberty. Associated congenital defects are common and include coarctation of the aorta and renal and skeletal anomalies. Laboratory analysis show absent barr body, 45 X chromosomal pattern and elevated plasma levels of gonadotrophins, particularly follicle stimulating hormone. The 45 X disorder occurs in approximately 1:3000 live female births. Mosaicism (46 XX/45 X) which is present in 25% of those with the syndrome has fewer and more attenuated abnormalities. The term 'Male Turner's syndrome' or Noonan's syndrome has been applied to phenotypic males who have certain anomalies which also occur in females with Turner's syndrome. The most common anomalies are short stature, webbing of the neck, congenital heart disease and a characteristic facies. They differ from true Turner's syndrome in that mental retardation is more common, they show a wide variety of gonadal defects and the cardiac defects are more often valvular in origin.

Vaughan V, McKay R, Behrmann R (eds) 1983 Nelson Textbook of Paediatrics 12th edn. Saunders, London
Pitcher D 1982 Sex chromosome disorders. In: Granville-Grossman K (ed) Recent Advances in Clinical Psychiatry. Churchill Livingstone, Edinburgh

31 Newly diagnosed cancer patients usually show shock and disbelief, occasional denial, anger, depression and suicidal ideation. These symptoms are seen as non-specific reactions to severe stress and it has been postulated that these symptoms signify a coping process leading to readjustment. With advanced cancer psychological distress is likely to occur either as a concomitant of the somatic sequelae such as pain, weakness and loss of bodily functions or because the lack of response to treatment signifies a long, lingering death to the patient. Neuropsychiatric symptoms may result from cerebral metastases, carcinomatous neuropathies and metabolic disturbances associated with the malignancy, such as hypercalcaemia. Some

40% of cancer patients referred for psychiatric opinion are noted to have an organic brain syndrome and significant depression is found in 20–25% of those with advanced cancer who are admitted to hospital. Of patients with pancreatic carcinoma 76% are found to be depressed and depression is the presenting feature in about one-half of cases. Psychological morbidity exists in long term survivors but the frequency and duration of the distress is not known. Radiotherapy, cytotoxic drugs and extensive surgery may each be followed by psychiatric symptoms. Treatment with radiotherapy or chemotherapy can lead to cognitive and affective symptoms. About 25% of women develop an affective illness within 18 months following mastectomy and other frequent sequelae include embarrassment with social isolation and marital and sexual difficulties. Similarly, depression, sexual problems and social isolation are noted frequently after colostomy.

Fras I, Lotin E M, Pearson J S 1967 Companion to psychiatric symptoms in carcinoma of the pancreas with those of other intra-abdominal neoplasms. American Journal of Psychiatry 123: 1553–1562

Greer S 1985 Cancer: Psychiatric aspects. In: Granville–Grossman K (ed) Recent Advances in Clinical Psychiatry 5. Churchill Livingstone, Edinburgh

Levine P, Silberfarb P, Lipowski Z 1978 Mental disorders in cancer patients: a study of 100 psychiatric referrals. Cancer 42: 1385–1391

32 Yes. Mild mental handicap without organic pathology is found mostly in lower working class families and is rare in middle or upper classes. Even with severe subnormality there is a slight predominance in the lower social classes. Sociologically orientated studies emphasise the relationship between social disadvantage and mental handicap. This disadvantage is often compounded by the parents' social incompetence, which is in turn related to their own IQ. Birch noted that there was an increased frequency of mental handicap in those from large families, poor housing, disrupted schooling, family disorganisation and poverty. It was also noted that the siblings of handicapped subjects were twelve times more likely to be mentally handicapped than that of a comparison population.

Birch H, Richardson S, Baird D, Horobin G, Illsley R 1970 Mental subnormality in the community: a clinical and epidemiological study. Williams and Wilkins, Baltimore

Taylor E, Bickness J 1986 The psychiatry of mental handicap. In: Hill P, Murray R, Thorley A (eds) Essentials of Postgraduate Psychiatry 2nd edn. Grune and Stratton, London

33 Hyperactivity of dopaminergic neurones has been postulated as an explanation for the development of some schizophrenic symptoms. Amphetamines, which are known to produce a schizophrenic-like disorder, are thought to act by releasing dopamine and noradrenaline into the synaptic cleft and preventing their inactivation. Also, neuroleptic drugs have the ability to suppress transmission in central dopaminergic neurones. The degree of binding to dopamine receptors shows a significant positive correlation with the therapeutic effect of the neuroleptics and with the occurrence of Parkinson-like symptoms. The extrapyramidal side effects seem to be due to a functional dopamine deficiency in the nigro-striatal pathway. Johnstone demonstrated that the anti-psychotic effects of the neuroleptics was due to dopamine receptor blockade by comparing the cis- and trans-isomer of flupenthixol. Only the cis showed significant anti-psychotic action supporting the view that clinical efficiency depends on dopamine blockade. However, there is little direct evidence that simply over-activity of central dopaminergic neurones underlies the symptomatology. Plasma prolactin concentrations, which fall in response to high levels of dopamine, are not lowered in patients with the illness. In untreated schizophrenics dopamine metabolites in cerebrospinal fluid are not increased and post-mortem findings do not show any consistent evidence of increased dopamine release.

Johnstone E C, Crow T J, Frith C D, Carney M P W, Price J S 1978 Mechanisms of the antipsychotic effect in the treatment of schizophrenia. Lancet 1: 848–851

Van Praag H M 1986 The significance of dopamine for the mode of actions of neuroleptics and the pathogenesis of schizophrenia. In: Kerr A, Snaith P (eds) Contemporary Issues in Schizophrenia. Gaskell Psychiatry Series

34 This is a clinical neurological test which is useful for distinguishing between organic and functional psychiatric disorders. When light touch stimuli

are applied simultaneously to the cheek and hand patients with brain damage often only feel one of the stimuli or mislocate the more peripheral of the stimuli. Unlike a focal parietal lobe lesion, the extinction is present on both sides of the body. Normal subjects and patients with functional disorders might not detect or may mislocate one of the stimuli on the first few trials, but after 10 attempts almost all will be able to distinguish correctly between the stimuli, while 90% of patients with brain damage will continue to make errors of extinction or displacement.

Irving G, Robinson R A, McAdam W 1970 The validity of some cognitive tests in the diagnosis of dementia. British Journal of Psychiatry 117: 149–156

35 This is considered to be present when there is a sudden or severe change in a person's behaviour or emotions, due to an abnormal mental state sufficient to cause distress for the person in question, his family or the community. Such changes, if left unchecked, can result in suicide, panic attacks, crippling distress, impaired decision making, homicide or destruction of property. In practice an emergency exists when the patient or family perceive it to be present and their sense of urgency, which reflects an inability to cope, must be respected.

Urbaitis J C 1983 Definitions and basic concepts. In: Psychiatric Emergencies. Appleton-Century-Crofts, Norwalk, Connecticut

36 This is a 47 XXY karyotype abnormality which occurs in approximately one in every thousand live male births and it presents with varying degrees of gynaecomastia, small testes, sterility and eunuchoid body build. Mental subnormality, usually of a mild degree, is a common feature but many cases are within the normal range of intelligence. Speech, language and reading difficulties may be the most obvious features of the syndrome before puberty. There is an increased likelihood of developing psychiatric conditions, particularly personality and neurotic disorders. Laboratory investigations show that they are chromatin positive males with low plasma testosterone levels and testicular biopsy reveals azospermia, hyalinization of the seminiferous tubular membranes and clumping of Leydig cells. Those with a mosaic

pattern have lesser degrees of the clinical features while variants of the syndrome with increasing numbers of X chromosomes have more marked virilization and intellectual retardation.

Carter C O 1973 An ABC of Medical Genetics. Lancet, London

Murray R M, McGuffin P 1988 Genetic aspects of mental disorders. In: Kendell R E, Zealley A K (eds) Companion to Psychiatric Studies, 4th edn. Churchill Livingstone, Edinburgh

Nelson Textbook of Paediatrics 1983 Vaughan V, McKay R, Behrmann R (eds) Saunders, London

37   This is a subjective sensation of restlessness most often experienced in the legs and is one of the extrapyramidal side effects associated with phenothiazines. It is more marked when the person is sitting and is not distracted. The subject will pace incessantly, change the position of his feet or rock to and fro to lessen the sensation. It is most frequently encountered with the piperazine group of phenothiazines and is thought to result from an imbalance between dopamine and acetylcholine activity in the nigrostriatal system.

Silverstone T, Turner P 1982 Schizophrenia. In: Drug Treatment in Psychiatry 3rd edn. Routledge and Kegan Paul, London

38   The slow wave activity which occurs immediately following ECT tends to become more persistent with further treatments, but there is quite a degree of variability between subjects. After four ECTs, separated by 2–3 days, the slow wave activity remains and becomes of higher amplitude and lower frequency predominately in the frontal lobes, while alpha rhythm disappears with further treatments. These changes tend to correlate with the degree of confusion associated with treatment and they begin to revert to the pretreatment pattern 7–9 weeks after the last ECT.

Kiloh L G, McComas A J, Osselton J W 1979 Psychiatry. In: Clinical Electroencephalography 3rd edn. Butterworth, London

39   The practical aspects of immediate management of the patient stems directly from the evaluation of risk of suicide. High risk patients should be hospitalised immediately for their own protection and treatment. The decision whether to admit to hospital or not depends on the diagnosis and

severity of the psychiatric disorder, the patient's previous psychiatric history, the availability of social support and the presence or absence of other risk factors. Within the hospital setting a careful diagnostic evaluation should be done and where major psychiatric disorders, particularly depression exist, treatment should be instituted without delay. This usually consists of ECT or antidepressant medication in appropriate dosage. The level of supervision required by the suicidal patient should be clearly identified and re-evaluated frequently. Follow up planning should begin in hospital with evaluation of the family and social situation, establishment of a supportive therapeutic relationship and attention paid to well recognised risk factors such as loss and social isolation. Out-patient or day patient management may involve establishment of links with the social services, involvement of family and careful prescribing of psychotropic medication. Preferably a family member may take charge of the patient's drugs and these should be prescribed in small amounts. Evaluation and management of risk factors is paramount. Long term follow up by the family doctor, psychiatric or social services may follow.

Kreitman N 1988 Suicide and parasuicide. In: Kendell R E, Zealley A K (eds) Companion to Psychiatric Studies, 4th edn. Churchill Livingstone, Edinburgh
Morgan H G 1982 Deliberate self-harm. In: Granville–Grossman K (ed) Recent Advances in Clinical Psychiatry 4. Churchill Livingstone, Edinburgh

40 The aim is to encourage appropriate independent behaviour in the demented patient for as long as possible. Stimulation and activity programmes are designed to re-socialise people and improve their self esteem. Changes in the environment such as altering sitting arrangements and providing small living units for accommodation, rather than dormitories, may increase social interaction. Reality orientation therapy is a technique for teaching demented patients simple facts about time, place and persons around them and the names and uses of commonly used objects. It is widely practised in long term care facilities but there is little evidence of dramatic results in senile dementia. Much of the value of reality orientation may centre around the promotion of rapport between patients and therapeutic optimism among

the staff. Behavioural approaches have been applied to many situations such as eating, mobility, social interaction, participation in activities, incontinence and general hygiene. Many of these approaches are used in long stay residential care and day hospitals. At home, families can practise reality orientation and encourage use of domestic and social skills. A problem solving approach to these people is often adopted, such as use of diaries, clocks and following a structured routine. Supportive psychotherapy is very important for the patients, staff in hospitals and community services and the families of the elderly dementia patient.

Gurland B, Birkett D 1983 The senile and presenile dementias. In: Lader M (ed) Handbook of Psychiatry 2. Mental disorders and somatic illness. Cambridge University Press, Cambridge
Hussain R A 1981 Geriatric psychology: A behavioural perspective. Van Nostrand Reinhold, New York

41 Estimates of blood or urinary alcohol are helpful especially if elevated in the morning. Macrocytosis without anaemia occurs in some 80% and this is related to alcohol induced impairment of folate utilisation or low dietary folate intake. Liver function tests may show elevated serum levels of gamma glutamyl transpeptidase and alkaline phosphatase with low serum albumin. Liver biopsy is helpful in detecting alcohol induced hepatocellular damage. A proportion of alcoholics have evidence of hypomagnesaemia, hyperlipidaemia and hyperuricaemia and others are deficient in Vitamin B12 and folic acid.

Murray R, Bennadt M 1980 Early detection of alcoholism. Medical Education International Ltd 1108–1111
Ritson E B, Chick J 1988 Dependence on alcohol and other drugs. In: Kendell R E, Zealley A K (eds) Companion to Psychiatric Studies, 4th edn. Churchill Livingstone, Edinburgh

42 These drugs are dangerous in overdose, have a tendency to produce drug dependence and can induce hepatic microsomal enzymes. Initially barbiturates have a central excitatory effect which is followed by a depressant effect and in high doses they produce ataxia, confusion, stupor and unconsciousness. As little tolerance develops to the respiratory depressant effect, the chronic user

is particularly liable to have a respiratory arrest with overdoses. Drug dependency is manifested by a withdrawal syndrome characterised by agitation, psychotic delirium and grand mal seizures. Induction of hepatic microsomal enzymes reduces the half lives of such drugs; coumarin anticoagulants, griseofulvin, corticosteroids, phenytoin and oral contraceptives.

Silverstone T, Turner P 1982 (eds) Drug Treatment in Psychiatry 3rd edn. Routledge & Kegan Paul, London

43 They may occur as a result of any psychotic disturbance, organic brain disorder, suggestion, sensory deprivation, disorders of sense organs and be drug induced. A variety of organic states are associated with perceptual disturbance and any major disruption of cerebral function can produce hallucinations usually in association with clouding of consciousness. These organic states might result from metabolic and endocrine disorder, epilepsy, inflammatory or neoplastic disease or be drug related. Hallucinations may occur in schizophrenia, mania, depressive states and alcohol and drug withdrawal states. Hypnagogic and hypnopompic hallucinations can be regarded as special varieties of organic hallucinations. Hypnagogic hallucinations occur when the subject is falling asleep and hypnopompic when the subject is waking up. Hallucinatory voices may occur in ear disease or visual hallucinations in eye disease. Sensory deprivation may cause visual and auditory hallucinations, as is encountered in the delirium that occasionally follows cataract operations. Hallucinatory drugs induce a wide range of perceptual disturbances, chiefly visual phenomena. Several experiments have demonstrated that normal subjects can be persuaded to hallucinate either by suggestion alone, under hypnosis or by brief task-motivating instructions.

Mullen P E 1986 The mental state and states of mind. In: Hill P, Murray R, Thorley A (eds) Essentials of Postgraduate Psychiatry 2nd edn. Grune and Stratton, London

44 Yes. The whole range of psychiatric disorders is similar to that found in normal children. However, brain lesions are associated with an increased vulnerability to psychiatric disorders. In

the Isle of Wight study 50% of the severely retarded children were judged to have a psychiatric disorder as compared with 7% of children in the normal intelligence range. As in the general population of children of the same age, neurotic and conduct disorders were the most common, followed by mixed disorders with both emotional and antisocial features. However, certain disorders and particular items of behaviour are more common in the severely retarded group. Childhood psychoses, hyperkinetic behaviour disorder and isolated symptoms such as pica, self-injurious behaviour and severe stereotypes are relatively more frequent than in those with normal intelligence.

Corbett J 1985 Mental retardation: Psychiatric aspects. In: Rutter M, Hersov L (eds) Child and Adolescent Psychiatry 2nd edn. Blackwell, Oxford

Rutter M, Tizard J, Yule W, Graham P, Whitmore K 1976 Isle of Wight Studies 1964–1974. Psychological Medicine 6: 313–332

45 Kurt Schneider described a number of symptoms of the first rank which he considered to be diagnostic of schizophrenia in the absence of overt brain disease. These include auditory hallucinations taking one of three specific forms: voices repeating the subject's thoughts aloud, two or more hallucinatory voices arguing about or discussing the patient and referring to him in the third person, and voices commenting on the patient's thoughts or behaviour. Passivity phenomena include thought insertion, withdrawal or broadcast, feelings of the patient's body being influenced by outside sources and that emotions, drives and intentions are dictated by external forces. Primary delusions are also first rank symptoms. Criticism of Schneider's phenomenological approach is that 20% of chronic schizophrenics never show these symptoms and 8% of psychotic patients, who do not have schizophrenia, show these symptoms. Several studies have demonstrated that the symptoms have little prognostic significance.

Leff J 1982 Acute syndromes of schizophrenia. In: Wing J, Wing L (eds) Handbook of Psychiatry 3: Psychoses of uncertain aetiology. Cambridge University Press, Cambridge

Mellor C S 1982 The present status of first rank symptoms. British Journal of Psychiatry 140: 423–424

46 Most recent studies indicate that hysterectomy rarely leads to psychiatric disorder and that a history of pre-operative psychiatric disorder is one of the major determinants of post-operative functional illness. A neurotic personality, a positive psychiatric history and current psychiatric morbidity are the main predictors of psychiatric illness after hysterectomy. Impaired sexual functioning rarely results from hysterectomy in itself though major surgical resection may impair sexual activity through discomfort or pain.

Gath D, Cooper P, Day A 1981 (a) Hysterectomy and psychiatric disorder: Levels of psychiatric morbidity before and after hysterectomy. British Journal of Psychiatry 140: 335–342

Gath D, Cooper P 1982 Psychiatric aspects of hysterectomy and female sterilization. In: Granville–Grossman K (ed) Recent Advances in Clinical Psychiatry. Churchill Livingstone, Edinburgh

47 Widowed people, particularly elderly men, have an increased risk of suicide compared with an age and sex matched married population. The relative risk of suicide was estimated to be 2.5 times higher in the first year of bereavement and 1.5 times higher in the following three years. Bereaved people who committed suicide have significantly more psychiatric treatment and are more likely to have made a previous suicide attempt prior to the bereavement. Shepherd and Barraclough have shown that spouses of people who commit suicide do not have an increased mortality in the first year of bereavement, but follow-up studies of survivors of people who commit suicide show them to have a higher risk of death than survivors of other deaths.

Bunch J 1972 Recent bereavement in relation to suicide. Journal of Psychosomatic Research 16: 361–366

Shepherd D, Barraclough B M 1974 The aftermath of suicide. British Medical Journal 2: 600–603

48 The main tell-tale signs of abuse are a characteristic smell, glue on the hands and a facial rash. Initially after inhalation there is an excitatory phase followed by a depressive phase. This excitatory phase with feelings of euphoria, disinhibition, poor judgement, hallucinations and bizarre behaviour is fairly similar to the effects of alcohol, but toluene produces a quicker and briefer in-

toxication and more perceptual abnormalities. Recovery from the effects of inhalation follows within one hour with some degree of amnesia for the period. Other symptoms include sneezing, vomiting, tinnitus, blurred vision and lethargy. The central nervous system depressant effect may be severe and include disorientation, dysarthria, tinnitus, ataxia and nystagmus. These signs may progress to epileptic convulsions and coma. Deaths from asphyxia, laryngeal spasms and cardiac arrythmias have been reported. Blood levels of toluene are related to the severity of the clinical signs. Tolerance and withdrawal symptoms have been reported. Haematological abnormalities such as aplastic anaemia, eosinophilia and renal abnormalities have been described. Persistent neurological abnormalities have been attributed to toluene and other volatile substances and a cerebellar syndrome is the most common disorder being reported. Toluene may cause optic neuropathy and sensori-neural deafness in isolated cases, but its potential for causing peripheral neuropathy is low. Volatile substances such as N-hexane can cause peripheral neuropathy, but these substances are no longer present in the commonly used adhesives. There is some indication that structural brain changes may occur in chronic long term abusers. Psychiatric morbidity is high among abusers but there is little evidence to suggest that persistent or specific psychiatric disabilities result directly from sniffing glue.

Gordon A M 1985 Psychological aspects of drug abuse. In: Granville–Grossman K (ed) Recent Advances in Clinical Psychiatry. Churchill Livingstone, Edinburgh

Ron Maria A 1986 Volatile substance abuse. A review of possible long term neurological intellectual and psychiatric sequelae. British Journal of Psychiatry 148:, 235–247

49 This refers to children who have an underlying school refusal disorder which assumes a 'somatic disguise'. The complaints generally are of anorexia, nausea, vomiting, diarrhoea, abdominal pain, lightheadedness, vague pains and aches, weakness and palpitations. These symptoms occur in the morning before school or when at school, without any overt fear being expressed and the phobia is only elicited by careful enquiry. At times the somatic complaints are not experienced

but fearfully anticipated, so that the child avoids school in case he might faint or vomit.

Waller D, Eisenberg L 1980 School refusal in childhood—a psychiatric/paediatric perspective. In: Hersov L, Berg I (eds) Out of School. Wiley, Chichester

50 Parasuicide occurs predominantly among those aged 15–25 years. Females have higher rates with the overall female:male ratio usually being in the range of 1.4:1 to 2.2:1. Divorced people carry the greatest risk with single men of all ages showing higher rates than married men. Exceptionally high rates of parasuicide have been found in teenagers and single men over 35 years of age. Social classes IV and V show an increased incidence of deliberate self harm. A strong positive association exists between the incidence of deliberate self harm and areas of poor housing, overcrowding and few facilities. Other correlates include unemployment, marital disharmony, early parental loss, previous criminal record in males and families containing abused and 'at risk' children. Approximately 12% show psychotic illnesses, chiefly depressive or organic disorders and frequently alcohol abuse is implicated. Life event studies show that patients who harm themselves have an average of four times greater life event rate than expected, and some 50% show disruption in interpersonal relationships. Cultural attitudes within high risk areas enhance the likelihood of parasuicide.

Kreitman N 1988 Suicide and parasuicide. In: Kendell R E, Zealley A K (eds) Companion to Psychiatric Studies, 4th edn. Churchill Livingstone, Edinburgh

Morgan H G 1980 Social correlates of non-fatal deliberate self-harm. In: Farmer R D T, Hirsch S R (eds) The Suicide Syndrome. Croom Helm, London

51 Manic patients are usually brought along for treatment by relatives, concerned neighbours or the police and they rarely come of their own accord. They may appear to be relaxed and composed and not necessarily over-active in the formality of a doctor's surgery or emergency room, while the accompanying relative is often distressed by the disturbed behaviour. The first step in management is not to overlook the diagnosis or underestimate the extent of the mania; due regard must be given to the relatives' account. Given the

serious behavioural manifestations of mania, such as reckless driving and excessive spending, admission to hospital may be necessary until the patient's mood has been stabilised. This is even more necessary if the family are unable to manage the patient. Simple explanations should be given to the patient about the need for therapeutic intervention and while it is appropriate to repeat the explanation, it should be kept brief. If the patient is unwilling to co-operate with treatment and refuses to accept hospitalisation, having taken the necessary medicolegal steps, treatment should be administered with the assistance of adequate nursing personnel. Manic patients frequently make impossible demands and although they will verbally refuse to comply with medical recommendations, they will often accept these when they know the doctor is in control of the situation. In the acute emergency haloperidol should be administered intravenously, possibly along with an oral or intramuscular sedative phenothiazine such as chlorpromazine, until the mania is brought under control. It is probably best to give an anticholinergic drug simultaneously, in the initial stage, rather than wait for extrapyramidal side effects. The patient should be nursed in a low stimulus environment.

Urbaitis J C 1983 Psychosis. In: Psychiatric Emergencies. Appleton-Century-Crofts, Norwalk, Connecticut

52 The psychiatrist is involved in diagnosis, assessment, treatment and prevention of psychiatric disorders in physically ill patients and advises on psychological aspects of care of the physically ill. The psychiatrist also assesses and manages psychopathological reactions to organic illness, such as post-operative psychoses, paranoid states or hysterical reactions and is involved in the diagnosis and management of organic brain syndromes. These include alcohol and drug related states, confusional states in the elderly and psychological manifestations of endocrinopathies, neurological disorders and malignant disease. Being able to offer advice and support to the families of the physically ill, both directly and through medical and nursing staff, and attempting to prevent deviant illness behaviour consequent to physical illness are important aspects of his function. Special problems that may fall within the domain of the liaison psychiatrist include the management

of intractable pain and anorexia nervosa and the
assessment of suicidal risk, stupor and mutism.
He offers support to patients who are dying and
to their families and facilitates adequate communication between staff and patients, and supports
staff, both medical and non-medical, particularly
in intensive care, dialysis and oncology units.

Gelder M, Gath D, Mayou R 1983 (eds) Oxford
    Textbook of Psychiatry. Oxford University Press,
    Oxford
Gomez J 1981 Liaison psychiatry. British Journal
    Hospital Medicine, November, 1981 26: 242–246

53 Cognitive therapy is mainly used in depressive
states, eating disorders and anxiety neurosis.
Several trials provide strong evidence that cognitive therapy produces improvement in depression
of moderate severity, comparable to that produced
by antidepressant medication. However, it has not
been established that the effect is specific. The
cognitive approach to anxiety states is generally
a combination of explanation of the physiological
basis of anxiety, distraction, identification of the
anxiety provoking cognitions and teaching more
appropriate and alternative statements. These
techniques are generally combined with relaxation
therapy and other behavioural approaches. While
it is frequently used, its efficacy has not been
proven. A cognitive approach is gaining wide
acceptance in treating bulimia nervosa, but its
long term efficacy remains uncertain. Cognitive
therapy has also been used in anorexia nervosa
and obesity but the results are equivocal. Cognitive therapy, particularly in the form of problem
solving techniques, has been applied to a wide
variety of problems such as redundancy, divorce,
bereavement, pain, obsessional states and
alcoholism. However, its scientific value and
relevance to these clinical problems has yet to be
established.

Fairburn C G 1984 A cognitive behavioural treatment
    for bulimia. In: Garner D M, Garfinkel P E (ed)
    Handbook on Psychotherapy for Anorexia Nervosa
    and Bulimia. Guilford Press, New York
Gelder M 1985 Cognitive therapy. In:
    Granville–Grossman K (ed) Recent Advances in
    Clinical Psychiatry 5. Churchill Livingstone,
    Edinburgh
Murphy G, Simons A, Wetzel R, Lustman P 1984
    Cognitive therapy and pharmacotherapy: Singly and
    together in the treatment of depression. Archives of
    General Psychiatry 41: 33–41

54   The diagnosis should be considered where there
is a distinct deterioration of intellectual and social
functioning without any organic cause or where
new, bizarre, or unpredictable behaviour emerges.
The clinical picture is especially characterised by
poverty of thought. Delusions are less elaborate
than in the schizophrenia of those with normal
intelligence, while hallucinations are more primi-
tive and monotonous in type. Both these
phenomena may be identified more by the
patient's behaviour rather than · by verbal
communication. Prominent catatonic symptoms
may be present but must be distinguished from
stereotypies and mannerisms which may occur in
the retarded person. It is particularly difficult to
make a definitive diagnosis if the IQ is less than
50.

Taylor E, Bickness J 1986 The psychiatry of mental
handicap. In: Hill P, Murray R, Thorley A (eds)
Essentials of Postgraduate Psychiatry. Grune and
Stratton, London

55   Where the illness is mild, treatment can be given
at home but with extreme self-neglect, poor
compliance with medication, or marked degrees
of social disturbance admission to hospital will be
necessary. Frequently, patients lose their current
symptoms when transferred to hospital. The
response to phenothiazines is usually good. It is
preferable to use a phenothiazine with as few side
effects as possible. Thioridazine is recommended
but if relatively high doses fail to produce a useful
remission, more strongly antidopaminergic preparations, such as trifluoperazine or haloperidol,
may be needed. Depot medication may be recommended if the patient shows poor compliance.
Aggravating factors such as deafness should be
attended to. Approximately one-third of patients
show a complete remission of symptoms, one-
third will have fluctuating paranoid symptoms but
a quarter, despite initial response, will have a poor
outcome. The prognosis over a three year follow-
up is closely related to the maintenance of drug
therapy. Severe deafness, the presence of organic
cerebral disorder, a poor past personal adjustment
and lack of response to drugs are unfavourable
prognostic factors.

Jacoby R, Bergmann K 1986 The psychiatry of old
age. In: Hill P, Murray R, Thorley A (eds)
Essentials of Postgraduate Psychiatry, 2nd edn.
Grune and Stratton, London

Post F 1966 Persistent persecutory states of the
elderly. Pergamon Press, Oxford

56 Dementia refers both to specific diseases and to
a syndrome. As a clinical syndrome it is best
defined as an acquired global impairment of intellect, memory and personality, without disturbance
of consciousness. Usually it is a chronic,
progressive disorder and is frequently irreversible,
although these are not necessary aspects of the
syndrome as, for example, when it is due to B12
deficiency or a meningioma. As disease entities the
dementias refer to a specific group of disorders
known as the senile and presenile dementias.

Cutting J, McClelland R 1986 Psychiatric
manifestations of organic illness. In: Hill P, Murray
R, Thorley A (eds) Essentials of Postgraduate
Psychiatry. Grune and Stratton, London

57 The contraindications are: raised intracranial
pressure, suspected space occupying lesion in the
posterior fossa or in the supratentorial region,
ventricular dilation with suspected raised intracranial pressure and tissue suppuration at the
lumbar puncture site.

Weiner H L, Levitt L P 1983 Lumbar Puncture. In:
Neurology for House Officer 3rd edn. Williams and
Wilkins, Baltimore

58 Miles concluded that nearly all suicides in the
USA could be attributed to psychiatric disorder.
Barraclough estimated that 93% were psychiatrically ill at the time of the suicide. The incidence
of previous psychiatric contact in suicides has
been estimated at 50%. Depressive illness is associated with the highest suicide risk, and the risk
is twenty-five times greater than that in the
general population. Alcoholism and drug addiction are associated with an increased suicide risk
the rates being 75 and 20 times greater, respectively, than in the general population respectively. Approximately 15% of patients with depressive illness, 6–10% of hospitalised alcoholics and
10% of schizophrenics commit suicide. Evidence
of long standing personality difficulties may be
found in up to 50% of suicides. Miles estimated
that 5% of psychopathic patients will commit
suicide. Patients with neuroses also have an increased risk of suicide.

Roy A 1986 Self-destructive behaviour. In: Hill P,
Murray R, Thorley A (eds) Essentials of Postgraduate
Psychiatry, 2nd edn. Grune and Stratton, London.

59 The results of treatment are generally good. Prognosis depends on the severity of the disorder, the age of the child, the time between the onset of symptoms and beginning of treatment, and the stability of the family. A three-year follow up study indicated that approximately one-half to two-thirds of children successfully return to school, about one-third still have severe neurotic symptoms with social impairment and another third retain less disabling symptoms of emotional disturbance. Ten years later about 20% show persistent emotional disorder and social impairment. Agoraphobia in adult life may be preceded by school refusal in childhood. Berg and his colleagues noted that approximately one-third of adolescent school refusers may be expected to continue suffering from neurotic symptoms and social impairment in young adult life, though only a minority become agoraphobic.

Berg I, Rutter A, Hall G 1976 The outcome of adolescent school phobia. British Journal of Psychiatry 128: 80–85

Berg I 1982 When truants and school refusers grow up. British Journal of Psychiatry 141: 208–210

Tyrer P, Tyrer S 1974 School refusal, truancy and adult neurotic illness. Psychological Medicine 4: 416–421

60 The principal treatment methods are medication, psychological therapy and social therapy, which all interact in the rehabilitation process. Antipsychotic medication has been shown to be more effective than placebo in preventing relapse. Maintenance phenothiazine therapy has a protective effect in patients living with relatives where there is high expressed emotion and may also be of benefit to patients who may be exposed to stressful life events. The minimum effective level is the optimum regime as side-effects, such as weight gain, Parkinsonism and tardive dyskinesia, can be particularly disabling and they can result in poor drug compliance. Psychological therapy includes social skills training and behavioural techniques to improve self-care, lessen aggressive behaviour and promote social interaction. Occupational therapy concentrates on activities of daily living, social activities, handicrafts, budgeting and general household duties. Work, even in a sheltered setting, has an important role in rehabilitation. Work may range from industrial therapy in

hospital based units, through local authority sheltered workshops, to open employment. Because of the economic climate most schizophrenics are unemployed. Social work intervention helps the patient on practical problems, organising accommodation to suit the patient's needs and that of the family, and provides support for the patient and his family. Family therapy aims at supporting the family and reducing high expressed emotion. While the rehabilitation team may have access to a wide variety of techniques, each programme for the individual is decided through a thorough assessment of the patient.

Bebbington P, Kuipers L 1982 Social management of schizophrenia. British Journal of Hospital Medicine October 1982: 96–102

McCreadie R G 1986 Rehabilitation. In: Kerr A, Snaith P (eds) Contemporary Issues in Schizophrenia. Gaskell Psychiatry Series

61 These are ways of thinking that increase the possibility of unwarranted negative interpretations. Beck has described four types of distortion, or errors in logic. Selective abstraction is taking one or more details out of context and so producing a negative view of oneself. For example, a person is at a party and all but one friend greets him warmly; the patient sees himself as being a boring person. Arbitary inference is the process of interpreting a single event as evidence of failure or rejection without considering alternatives. One particular aspect of a patient's work is criticised so the patient concludes that all his work is incompetent. Over-generalisation means making a general conclusion based on one incident, e.g. a woman that spoils a dinner feels she is a totally useless person. Magnification he describes as interpreting a minor problem as a major disaster and minimization refers to the process of undervaluing one's achievements. These errors are central to the salient theories of depression—self-blame, deprecatory feelings, helplessness and hopelessness.

Goddard A 1982 Cognitive behaviour therapy and depression. British Journal of Hospital Medicine March: 248–250

62 There is little evidence that pure opiates directly cause physical damage. The high morbidity and

mortality seem to be related to the lifestyle of the addict, his physical and social neglect and the use of contaminated drugs and needles. Addicts have a high incidence of hepatitis and abnormal liver function tests, but these abnormalities are possibly directly related to injecting habits. Septic complications occur in 40%. Other complications include the nephrotic syndrome, endocarditis, tuberculosis, pulmonary oedema and angio-thrombotic pulmonary hypertension which is caused by embolization to the lung of inert filler material in capsules when its contents are injected intravenously. Death results from septicaemia, overdose, other physical complications, suicide and poly-drug abuse. The mortality rate among opiate addicts has been estimated to be 20–25 times greater than the expected rate for non-drug dependent individuals and it varies from 16–30 per 1,000 addicts per year in the USA and Britain.

Grimes J A 1977 Drug dependence study. A survey of drug addicts attending for treatment. Statistics and Research Division, DHSS, London

Thorley A 1986 Drug problems. In: Hill P, Murray R, Thorley A (eds) Essentials of Postgraduate Psychiatry 2nd edn. Grune and Stratton, London

63 Earlier studies indicated that there were two types of abnormal grief reactions: delayed or avoided grief and chronic grief. Chronic grief is defined as an abnormal prolongation and intensification of the typical grief pattern. Delayed grief is a mixed form in which a typical or chronic reaction takes place after a period of delay during which the full expression of grief is inhibited. Parkes and Weiss have more recently elaborated three common patterns of pathological grief. In the unexpected grief syndrome which follows unexpected major losses, the initial disbelief and denial persists for a longer period with marked anxiety symptoms before the full emotional reaction is experienced. In the ambivalent grief syndrome where the relationship with the deceased was one of ambivalence, the immediate reaction is relief. Later feelings of intense despair and self-punitive behaviour may be severe and prolonged. These two types account for most of the delayed griefs seen in clinical practise. In chronic grief the reaction is typical but continues for an abnormal length of time and usually reflects the very dependent relationship the bereaved had with the deceased.

These grief patterns may occur in either their pure form or in combination.

Murray C, Parkes C M 1965 Bereavement and mental illness, Part II. A classification of bereavement reactions. British Journal Medical Psychology 38: 13–26
Parkes C M, Weiss R 1983 Recovery from bereavement. Basic Books, New York

64 A favourable prognosis is associated with single marital status, high educational achievement, high socio-economic group, skilled or professional employment, early age of onset and early presentation, satisfactory parental relationships, good premorbid personality, over-activity and admission to feelings of hunger. The following factors usually indicate an unfavourable prognosis: poor premorbid personality as evinced by unsatisfactory relationships and relative psychosexual immaturity, purging and vomiting, bulimic episodes, severe weight loss, previous hospitalisation and a chronic course. Other poor prognostic indices include late age of onset, male sex, body image disturbance, denial of the illness and poor motivation for change, higher rates of physical complaints, marriage, parental conflict and parental psychiatric morbidity.

Psychological Medicine 1983 Editorial, Follow up studies of anorexia nervosa, 239–249

65 This syndrome is a rare and potentially lethal disorder occurring in 0–1% of patients taking neuroleptic medication. Its clinical features are characterised by muscular rigidity, akinesia, hyperthermia, autonomic instability and altered consciousness. Rhabdomyolysis may occur, resulting in high levels of creatinine phosphokinase and renal failure. Other complications include respiratory failure, myocardial infarction and hepatic failure. Laboratory data show non-specific changes only. Disorders to be considered in the differential diagnosis include severe dystonic reactions, malignant hyperthermia, allergic drug reactions, infections, toxic encephalopathies, akinetic mutism and catatonia. The pathogenesis underlying this syndrome is unclear but is thought to be related to blockade of hypothalamic dopamine receptors by neuroleptics or a direct toxic effect on skeletal muscle. Treatment

consists of drug withdrawal and supportive measures. Specific drug measures have had limited success. At present the most useful drugs appear to be a combination of dantrolene and bromocriptine. The syndrome has also been attributed to tetrabenazine and alpha methyl tyrosine and can follow the withdrawl of levodopa and amantidine.

Abbott R J, Loizou L A 1986 Neuroleptic malignant syndrome. British Journal of Psychiatry 148: 47–52
Levenson J 1985 Neuroleptic malignant syndrome. American Journal of Psychiatry 142: 1137–1146

66 Many different intelligence tests are in use, the two most common being the Wechsler Adult Intelligence Scale and the Wechsler Intelligence Scale for Children. These tests comprise of eleven sub-tests which test verbal and performance abilities. Other intelligence tests include the Stanford Binet Intelligence Scale, the Neville Palmer Scale and the British Ability Scales. For developmental assessment the Denver Scale or the Griffith's Mental Scale is used. The Griffith's Scale is probably more accurate and tests five fields of development: locomotion, social, speech, hand-eye and performance and practical reasoning abilities. It may be used from infancy to eight years. Social development is assessed by the Vineland Social Maturity Scale. This tests a wide range of skills and is suitable for unco-operative children. The Gunsburg Progress Assessment Charts record development under four headings: self-help, communication, socialisation and occupation. A number of skills are included under each heading and the charts allow easy visual comparison of those skills present on initial recording with those noted on subsequent occasions and helps to identify special weaknesses.

Taylor E, Bickness J 1986 The psychiatry of mental handicap. In: Hill P, Murray R, Thorley A (eds) Essentials of Postgraduate Psychiatry 2nd edn. Grune and Stratton, London

67 The main disorders to be considered include manic-depressive psychoses, reactive psychoses, schizo-affective disorder, paranoid psychoses and organic brain syndromes. Manic patients may present with over inclusive thinking and first rank symptoms as may patients with schizo-affective disorder. Occasionally obsessional neurosis will cause diagnostic confusion and here the distinc-

tion between an obsession and a delusion must be made. Several personality disorders need to be considered. Subjects with schizoid personality traits show an apparent lack of feeling, have few friends and are socially isolated, but lack psychotic symptoms. Paranoid personalities are generally rigid, suspicious and morbidly sensitive. Borderline personality disorders may present with 'micro psychotic' episodes precipitated by stressful events. Paranoid states such as morbid jealousy, paranoia, De Clerambault's syndrome and *folie à deux* need to be considered. Organic disorders which may mimic schizophrenia and may not be readily obvious include temporal lobe epilepsy, intracranial space occupying lesions, metabolic disorders and neurosyphilis. Most hallucinatory and stimulant drugs are capable of causing psychoses, chiefly amphetamine, alcohol, cocaine, cannabis, phencyclidine and LSD. Others include steroids, digoxin, procyclidine and other anti-cholinergic drugs and antihypertensive drugs. Neurological disorders which can be associated with a schizophrenic-like state include systemic lupus erythematosis, Huntington's chorea, Parkinson's disease, disseminated sclerosis, Wilson's disease and idiopathic calcification of the basal ganglia.

Doran A, Breier A, Roy A 1986 Differential diagnosis and diagnostic systems in schizophrenia. In: Roy A (ed) The Psychiatric Clinics of North America. Schizophrenia, 17–35. Saunders, Philadelphia
Murray R 1986 Schizophrenia. In: Hill P, Murray R, Thorley A (eds) Essentials of Postgraduate Psychiatry 2nd edn. Grune and Stratton, London

68 This syndrome applies to the physical and psycho-logical symptoms that occur before and during the menstrual period in females. Common physical symptoms include abdominal discomfort, breast tenderness, headaches, skin eruptions and a subjective feeling of swelling. Irritability, tension, anxiety, sleep disorder and depressed mood are the main psychological symptoms. The estimated frequency of these complaints range from 30–80%. A connection between psychotic disorders, whether affective, cognitive or mixed has been suggested. However, this association seems to result from a premenstrual exacerbation of concurrent psychiatric symptomatology. Clare demonstrated a significant association between premenstrual complaint and psychiatric morbidity

but found little evidence to support the view that the premenstrual disorder caused the psychiatric ill health. It seems more likely that psychiatric ill health and social stresses may aggravate normal premenstrual variations in mood and physical wellbeing.

Clare A 1983 Psychiatric and social aspects of premenstrual complaints. Psychological Medicine Monographic Supplement 4. Cambridge University Press, Cambridge

69 The most well established and extensively researched system for classifying depression is that of the endogenous-neurotic category. While there is a wealth of clinical, therapeutic, statistical and now laboratory evidence to support the concept of endogenous depression being a homogenous entity, the position of neurotic-reactive depression is less certain. The Research Diagnostic Criteria incorporates the endogenous-neurotic dichotomy, while the DSM III uses the term melancholia to refer to endogenous depression. Van Praag and his colleagues describe 'vital' depression in contrast to 'personal' depression which is situation based. Feighner proposed separating affective disorders into primary and secondary forms, primary being defined as depression or mania occurring in a patient without a previous history of another psychiatric diagnosis, and secondary as a depressive syndrome occurring with a pre-existing non-affective psychiatric illness or the concurrence of a life threatening or incapacitating medical illness. Recent surveys have indicated that the primary and secondary types do not differ in the treatment received, the therapeutic response nor in the rate of affective disorders detected among first degree relatives. Another classification proposed by Winokur is based on the observations that among primary depressives of the Feighner type early onset depressives contained more females than those of late onset and that the male relatives of early onset females had a higher prevalence of alcoholism and antisocial personality, while female relatives tended to have a higher rate of depression. On this basis, he has divided primary unipolar depressives into 'pure depressives' occurring typically in males over the age of 40 with a family history of depression, where male and female relatives have an equal prevalence of depression, 'depression spectrum disease' tending

to occur in young women with a family history of antisocial personality, alcoholism and affective disorder and finally the 'non-familial group' who have no family history of a major psychiatric disorder. The 'pure depressives' and the 'non-familial group' tend to have similar symptoms and a better response to antidepressant treatments than the 'depression spectrum disease' group who are more likely to benefit from major tranquillisers. The validity of this classification has not yet been fully explored.

Feighner J P, Robins E, Guze S B, Woodruff R A, Winokur G, Munoz R 1972 Diagnostic criteria for use in psychiatric research. Archives of General Psychiatry 26: 57–63

Winokur G 1979 Unipolar depression. Is it divisable into autonomous subtypes. Archives of General Psychiatry 36: 47–52

70 Management of opiate dependence involves making a detailed enquiry into the history of drug usage and assessing the addict's ongoing drug requirements, treating medical complications such as abscesses, infections, endocarditis and hepatitis and providing a long term rehabilitation programme. Initial hospitalisation of the addict allows the opportunity for a detailed history and physical examination, observation of withdrawal effects, urinalysis and screening for polydrug abuse, medical treatment of physical complications and provides an environment where a therapeutic relationship with staff can be established. Methadone is the drug of choice in treatment of the abstinence syndrome. Generally, when withdrawal signs are noted 10–20 mg of Methadone is administered and repeated when further withdrawal symptoms occur. After one to two days a daily stabilisation dose is calculated which is rarely in excess of 50 mgs and this should be reduced by approximately 5 mg each day. Narcotic antagonists such as naltrexone and cyclazocine has been used for treating opiate dependent patients, but the results of treatment are very variable. Acupuncture is occasionally used. Patients can be detoxified as in-patients or they can be stabilised as out-patients on a maintenance dose of methadone for a period of time. Methadone is prescribed in linctus or injectable form and should be dispensed on a daily basis. The dose is gradually reduced until abstinence is achieved. This is coupled with social and

occupational rehabilitation and attendance at day centres and residential therapeutic communities. Synanon, Phoenix House and similar houses provide an alternative drug free community for addicts. Narcotic Anonymous meetings which are based on the philosophy of Alcoholics Anonymous help to sustain abstinence.

DHSS 1982 Treatment and rehabilitation. Report of the Advisory Council on the misuse of drugs. Her Majesty's Stationery Office, London

DHSS 1984 Guidelines of good clinical practice in the treatment of drug misuse. Report on the Medical Working Party on drug dependence. DHSS, London

Thorley A 1983 a) Rehabilitation of problem drinkers and drug takers. In: Watts F, Bennett D H (eds) Psychiatric Rehabilitation in Theory and Practice. Wiley, Chichester

71   This term depicts the neurological cognitive and personality sequelae that appears to follow repeated mild head injury and has been described in boxers. The amount of damage is proportional to the number and strength of the concussion blows inflicted. Neurological features include dysarthria, poverty and clumsiness of movement, rigidity with Parkinsonian-type gait and tremor. Evidence of asymmetrical pyramidal lesions are common from an early stage and cerebellar and extrapyramidal signs eventually appear. Mild memory impairment may progress to severe dementia. Personality changes include paranoia and morbid jealousy, rage reactions, irritability, apathy and occasionally there may be psychotic features. Pathological nerve cell loss, neurofibrillary tangles, brain stem damage, cortical infarcts and haemorrhages and characteristic perforation of the septum pellucidum have been found at post-mortem.

Lishman W A 1978 (ed) Head injury. In: Organic Psychiatry. Blackwell, Oxford

72   Wernicke's encephalopathy, which is caused directly by thiamine deficiency, is most commonly encountered in alcoholism. It is more rarely associated with other disorders inducing thiamine depletion such as prolonged vomiting or diarrhoea, dietary deficiency and carcinoma of the stomach and rarely in instances of increased body

requirements such as hyperthyroidism, pregnancy, lactation and prolonged fever.

Lishman W A 1978 Vitamin deficiencies. In: Organic Psychiatry. Blackwell, Oxford

73 Most programmes represent a mixture of behavioural, cognitive and psychodynamic approaches. Education of the couple aims to eliminate sexual myths and provide information concerning sexual anatomy and usual responses. The 'sensate focus' or mutual pleasuring technique of Masters and Johnson, which is the basis of the behavioural component improves communication, increases a feeling of security and decreases performance anxiety. This involves the couple in caressing each other with a ban on sexual intercourse, in order to give enjoyment. Emphasis is placed on the experience of sensation rather than the immediate achievement of orgasm. Special techniques are devised for specific problems. The squeeze technique is used for premature ejaculation. Vaginismus may be treated by use of vibrators or alternatively by digital examination by the female and her partner. Females with orgasmic difficulties may need individual sessions consisting of exploratory self-examinations which concentrate on pleasurable components. 'Stimulation therapy' which involves the use of sexually arousing photographs and films has been recommended for patients with low levels of sexual drive. Social skills training, exchange of contracts and masturbatory training may also form part of a treatment programme. Dynamic psychotherapy which explores the unconscious determinants of the patient's behaviour may be used.

Frank O S 1982 The therapy of sexual dysfunction. Symposium on Sexual Dysfunction 140: 86–92
Masters W, Johnson V 1970 Human sexual inadequacy. Little Brown, Boston

74 Kinsey and his colleagues in a survey of white American males found that 10% had been more or less exclusively homosexual for at least three years between the ages of 16 and 45 years, and a third had had one homosexual experience to the point of orgasm since adolescence, but only 4% remained exclusively homosexual throughout their lives. Gagnon and Simon re-analysed Kinsey's data and suggested that 3% of adult males had

extensive bisexual histories and only 3% were exclusively homosexual. Hunt's survey found that 1% of males were homosexual and 1% were bisexual. In their survey of women, Kinsey noted a much lower incidence of homosexual activity than in men: a similar re-analysis of the figures by Gagnon and Simon showed that only 6% had at least one homosexual experience and less than 1% were exclusively homosexual. Overall, the incidence in European studies is lower and this may reflect a bias in Kinsey's sampling technique.

Gagnon J, Simon W 1973 Sexual conduct: The social sources of human sexuality. Aldine, Chicago

Kinsey A, Pomeroy W, Martin C 1948 Sexual behaviour in the human male. Saunders, Philadelphia

Kinsey A, Pomeroy W, Martin C, Gebhard P 1953 Sexual behaviour in the human female. Saunders, Philadelphia

75 The initial outcome is favourable, but longer follow-up studies have shown that only a minority make a lasting recovery. Post in (1972) a three year study showed that one-quarter had recovered well, another one-third had recovered well but had had one or more recurrences within the three year period, one-quarter had recurrent attacks in the setting of chronic mild depression and some 12% were continuously ill throughout the follow-up period. Three of eighty-one patients had committed suicide. Murphy (1983) in a one-year follow-up of depressed elderly people showed that 43% remained well and 57% either showed no recovery or suffered early relapses. In both studies there were no unequivocal indicators of prognosis. However, long duration of depressive symptomatology before treatment seemed to militate against a good outcome. Outcome also was influenced by concurrent cerebral and non-cerebral organic disease, a higher chronological age and lower social class. The class effect was thought to exert its influence through the number of adverse life events experienced. The possession of a confiding relationship was not protective once the depression was established.

Murphy E 1983 Prognosis of depression in old age. British Journal of Psychiatry 142: 111–119

Post F 1972 The management and nature of depressive illnesses in late life: A follow through study. British Journal of Psychiatry 121: 393–404

76   Tics are sudden brisk involuntary contractions of
individual groups of muscle. They are repetitive,
non-purposeful, usually rapid and transient in
nature. They are exacerbated by anxiety, can be
suppressed or reproduced voluntarily and they
disappear during sleep. The usual age of presentation is between five and ten years and tics show
a three-fold male predominance. The most
common forms are facial tics, such as blinks,
grimaces and throat clearing. Tics may spread to
cause jerking of the neck, trunk and limbs and
vocal tics occur in Gilles de la Tourette syndrome.
There is no association between IQ and general
tics. They must be distinguished from chorieform
movements, myoclonic jerks, dystonic movements, dyskinesias and hemiballismic movements.
Simple tics are generally treated with explanation
and reassurance and by asking the patient to
ignore them. With persisting tics a full psychiatric
assessment is required. Behavioural techniques
such as massed practice or contingency management have been advocated but their efficacy has
not been established. Treatment with haloperidol
is indicated in the more severe cases and pimozide
and clonidine have also been used.

Hill P 1986 Child psychiatry. In: Hill P, Murray R,
  Thorley A (eds) Essentials of Postgraduate
  Psychiatry 2nd Edn. Grune and Stratton, London
Shapiro A, Shapiro E 1981 The treatment and
  aetiology of tics and Tourette syndrome.
  Comprehensive Psychiatry 22: 193–205

77   Evidence for a genetic predisposition comes from
family, twin and adoption studies. The familial
clustering of schizophrenia is evidenced by the
fact that the life time expectancy of schizophrenia
is some ten times greater for the first degree relatives of patients with this diagnosis than it is for
the general population where the risk is about 1%.
The risk for the children when both parents are
schizophrenic is about 35%. The concordance rate
between monozygotic twins for this disorder is
between 35 and 60% and 10–25% for dizygotic
pairs. Gottesman and Shields found that for
monozygotic twins discordance was most common
when the proband had a mild non-nuclear illness
and was very uncommon where the index twin
had a severe chronic illness. The concordance
rates for monozygotic pairs are similar whether
the twins are reared together or apart. Heston and

Denney studied the adopted away children of schizophrenic mothers and found that the offspring were considerably more disordered, with 10% being diagnosed schizophrenic, compared to the children of controls, none of whom had schizophrenia. Kety and his colleagues found that 14% of the biological relatives of adoptees with schizophrenia had schizophrenic spectrum disease compared to 2.7% of the adoptive relatives. Furthermore, the rate of schizophrenia was not increased among the adoptive parents of children who developed schizophrenia in adult life, suggesting that the parent-child interaction may not be an important causative factor.

Fish F J 1984 Fish's schizophrenia 3rd edn. Hamilton M (ed) Wright, Bristol

Murray R, Reveley A 1986 Genetic aspects of schizophrenia: Overview. In: Kerr A, Snaith P (eds) Contemporary Issues in Schizophrenia. Gaskell Psychiatry Series

78 Yes. Research has demonstrated a close association between substance abuse, particularly alcohol and suicidal behaviour. Retrospective studies confirm that alcohol is second only to affective disorder among the psychiatric disorders associated with suicide and 15–30% of suicide victims have alcoholism. Approximately 6–10% of hospitalised alcoholics commit suicide. The suicide rate in alcoholism is estimated at 75 times that expected in the general population. Acute alcohol intoxication is very frequent at the time of suicide. Adverse life events such as loss of job or close relationship and males aged 45–65 are especially likely to commit suicide. Alcohol abuse is a common theme in parasuicide, both in the form of chronic problem drinking as well as recent intake prior to the act of self harm. A suicide rate twenty times that of the general population has been reported in British heroin addicts. They are more likely to commit suicide at an earlier age than alcoholics and compared to other diagnostic grouping under the age of 40 they have the highest suicide rate.

Galanter M, Castaneda R 1985 Self-destructive behaviour in the substance abuser. In: Roy A (ed) The Psychiatric Clinics of North America. Self-destructive behaviour, 251–263. Saunders, Philadelphia

79 Initially one should check on the patient's compliance with the neuroleptic drug, ensure that an adequate dosage is being prescribed and consider using an alternative neuroleptic. There is considerable variation within the individual in plasma steady state concentrations of different neuroleptics. When a patient fails to respond to one neuroleptic there might be pharmacokinetic as well as practical reasons for switching to another. There are varying reports of the efficacy of propranolol but its role is still uncertain. Recent work using low and high dose propranolol shows that it has no beneficial effect, but when combined with a neuroleptic its effect may be to increase the neuroleptic plasma levels rather than having any direct pharmacological action of its own. Lithium has been shown to have an anti-psychotic effect and it may be useful in schizophrenia, even if no affective symptoms are present. Reports suggest that up to 50% may show improvement by the addition of lithium. Carbamazepine has been recommended by some as a substitute for lithium while others see its use only if there is temporal lobe involvement or EEG abnormalities. Tricyclic antidepressants may be of benefit if there is a clear depressive disorder.

Morgan R 1985 Drug treatment in psychiatry. Chronic Schizophrenia. British Journal of Hospital Medicine 34 (4): 202–205

Zemlaw F, Hirschonowitz J, Sautter F, Garvey D 1984 Impact of lithium therapy in core psychiatric symptoms in schizophrenia. British Journal of Psychiatry 144: 64–69

80 'Therapeutic' or 'curative' factors are psychological processes that take place in groups which contribute to a patient's improvement and are functions of the actions of the therapist, other group members and the patient. Though the individual factors operate in every therapy group, their interplay may vary widely from group to group. Also, patients in the same group may benefit from widely differing clusters of curative factors. Yalom divided the factors into eleven primary categories: cohesiveness refers to the feeling of belonging to and acceptance by a group, interpersonal learning is learning from the successes and failures of others, universality is the ability to perceive that other members of the group have similar problems and feelings, the

altruistic factor refers to the patient feeling better about himself and learning something positive about himself through helping other members of the group. The corrective recapitulation of the primary family group means that early family conflicts are recapitulated by the group members but they are relived correctively. Other 'curative factors' include instillation of hope, imparting of information, development of socialising techniques, imitative behaviour and cathartic and existential factors.

Bloch S, Crouch E, Rebstein J 1981 Therapeutic factors in group psychotherapy: A review. Archives of General Psychiatry 38: 519–526

Yalom I 1975 (ed) The theory and practice of group psychotherapy, 2nd edn. Basic Books, New York

81   Sedative drugs such as barbiturates and to a lesser extent chloral, paraldehyde, meprobamate and the various benzodiazepines produce an increase in the amount of fast activity in the 20–30 Hz range, often up to an amplitude of 100 μv. There is considerable variation both in the direct effect of these drugs and in the indirect effect they produce through drowsiness. Major tranquillisers and tricyclic antidepressants have a similar effect; they increase the amount of alpha activity if it is scanty and decrease it when it is plentiful and may decrease the amount of fast activity. With higher doses generalised delta activity may occur. Hypersynchronous high voltage discharges occur on occasions and both drugs potentiate epileptiform discharges. These changes again vary greatly between individuals and the recordings revert to normal some 10 weeks following cessation of treatment. Lithium carbonate produces an increased frequency of slow wave activity with a decrease in alpha waves and an increase in the amplitude of the record. After a month of treatment chronic changes appear alongside the early features in the form of focal abnormalities and paroxysmal spike activity.

Kiloh L G, McComas A J, Osselton J W 1979 Psychiatry. In: Clinical Electroencephalography 3rd edn. Butterworth, London

82   The most well established and extensively researched system for classifying depression is that of the endogenous-neurotic category. While there is a wealth of clinical, therapeutic, statistical and now laboratory evidence to support the

concept of endogenous depression being a homogenous entity, the position of neurotic-reactive depression is less certain. The Research Diagnostic Criteria incorporates the endogenous-neurotic dichotomy, while the DSM III uses the term melancholia to refer to endogenous depression. Van Praag and his colleagues describe 'vital' depression in contrast to 'personal' depression which is situation based. Feighner proposed separating affective disorders into primary and secondary forms, primary being defined as depression or mania occurring in a patient without a previous history of another psychiatric diagnosis and secondary as a depressive syndrome occurring with a pre-existing non-affective psychiatric illness or the concurrence of a life threatening or incapacitating medical illness. Recent surveys indicate that the primary and secondary types do not differ in the treatment received, the therapeutic response and in the rate of affective disorders detected among first degree relatives. Another classification proposed by Winokur is based on the observations that among primary depressives of the Feighner type early onset depressives contained more females than those of late onset and that the male relatives of early onset females had a higher prevalence of alcoholism and antisocial personality, while female relatives tended to have a higher rate of depression. On this basis, he has divided primary unipolar depressives into 'pure depressives' occurring typically in males over the age of 40 with a family history of depression, where male and female relatives have an equal prevalence of depression, 'depression spectrum disease' tending to occur in young women with a family history of antisocial personality, alcoholism and affective disorder and finally the 'non-familial group' who have no family history of a major psychiatric disorder. The 'pure depressives' and the 'non-familial group' tend to have similar symptoms, have a better response to antidepressant treatments than the 'depression spectrum disease' who are more likely to benefit from major tranquillisers. The validity of this classification has not yet been fully explored.

Feighner J P, Robins E, Guze S B, Woodruff R A, Winokur G, Munoz R 1972 Diagnostic criteria for use in psychiatric research. Archives General Psychiatry 26: 57–63

Winokur G 1979 Unipolar depression. Is it divisable into autonomous subtypes. Archives General Psychiatry 36: 47–52

83 Bereavement is followed by an increased incidence of depressive and neurasthenic symptoms, including anorexia and weight loss, fatigue, poor sleep and impaired concentration. Clayton showed that a triad of depressed mood, disturbed sleep and tearfulness was seen in over 50% of their bereaved subjects and over one-third met criteria for depression at one month after death. She also noted a one year incidence figure of 47% for depressive syndrome in bereaved people compared to 8% in a control population. The full range of depressive symptoms is common in the first year, though morbid guilt, suicidal ideation after one month and psychomotor retardation are more indicative of pathological reactions. Most bereaved people accept their symptoms as part of a normal reaction to death and they usually report feeling better after one year. The largest proportion of bereaved psychiatric patients are classified as suffering from reactive depression and anxiety and are found to be suffering from pathological forms of grief. All studies emphasise the increased use of alcohol, tranquillisers and hypnotics in bereaved people. The rate of psychiatric referral is increased during the first year in the young individual who is widowed, but the likelihood of being hospitalised for a psychiatric disorder is not increased, and if this occurs the diagnosis is most likely to be alcoholism. The widowed have an increased suicide rate compared to an age and sex matched married population and this is particularly true of elderly men.

Clayton P S, Halikas J A, Maurice W L 1972 The depression and widowhood. British Journal of Psychiatry 120: 71–77

Clayton P S 1982 Bereavement. In: Paykel E S (ed) Handbook of Affective Disorders. Churchill Livingstone, Edinburgh

84 There are three main approaches used in treatment. Firstly, there are methods used to decrease sexual deviant interest and behaviour. These include aversive therapy using either electric shock, chemicals or shame, covert sensitisation and self-control techniques. Secondly, there are treatment techniques aimed at increasing non-deviant sexual interest and behaviour. These techniques include fantasy modification using orgasmic reconditioning, fantasy shaping and exposure to explicit stimuli, and operant and classical condition procedures such as shaping, fading, biofeed-

back, aversion relief and systematic desensitisation. Some patients with deviant preferences or their partners have sexual dysfunctions and treatment of these dysfunctions using Masters and Johnson approach may help decrease the deviant behaviour. Social skills training is also used to help establish rewarding heterosexual relationships. These two approaches should not usually be used in isolation as they are often unsuccessful when used alone and this is particularly so for aversion therapy. The third form of behaviour therapy is used to help people who do not want to abandon their deviant sexual activity but may need help adjusting to it. These approaches generally involve a programme of social skills training, modelling and rehearsal of appropriate gender role behaviour and self-control procedures.

Hawton K 1983 Behavioural approaches to the management of sexual deviations. British Journal of Psychiatry 143: 248–256

Kellett J, Bebbington P 1986 Sexual disorders. In: Hill P, Murray R, Thorley A (eds) Essentials of Postgraduate Psychiatry 2nd edn. Grune and Stratton, London

85 Brain damaged children have been shown to have a five-fold increase in psychiatric disorders when compared with a normal population and a three-fold increase over children with chronic physical illness not affecting the brain. While the pathogenesis of psychiatric disorders in mental handicap is poorly understood, it can be said that they are not linked genetically and that the psychiatric disorders do not cause the intellectual retardation. The extent and location of the brain damage seem to be the important determinants, especially in those with severe subnormality. They indirectly exert a further influence where they produce epilepsy, hyperkinetic syndrome, personality disorder and additional handicaps such as visual, hearing or speech difficulties. Adverse temperamental features include irritability, which is an early characteristic of the asphyxiated brain damaged infant, impairment of attention and concentration. The reactions of parents to a handicapped and difficult child may interfere with the early development of coping skills, by the stigmatising effect of the handicap and by the unwanted effects of anti-convulsant medication on cognition and behaviour. Educational failure has been implicated in antisocial behaviour, especially

when accompanied by unrealistic expectations. General family disruption, punitive styles of management and cold rejecting attitudes are strongly associated with conduct disorders.

Corbett J 1985 Mental retardation: Psychiatric aspects. In: Rutter M, Hersov L (eds) Child and Adolescent Psychiatry 2nd Edn. Blackwell, Oxford

86 This syndrome is characterised by abnormalities of cognition, language and social development with stereotyped behaviour and routines. Most of these children are mentally handicapped and their IQs are stable and do not increase with improved socialisation. Performance scores characteristically exceed verbal scores. Abnormalities of language and communication affect understanding and the use of non-verbal as well as verbal communication methods. Speech problems include mutism, which is present in about 50% of cases, immediate and delayed echolalia, repetitive and stereotyped use of speech, telegrammatic neologisms and in the most able of children a grammatical but inappropriate pedantic and concrete style of expression. Pronoun reversal and a peculiar, idiosyncratic use of words and phrases is characteristic. Impairments occur in social interaction, communication and imagination. These problems include an aloofness and indifference to people, poor gaze contact, lack of curiosity, insensitivity to people's feelings and lack of awareness of social conventions. Those children form weak parental bonds and have no persisting relationships. They tend to indulge in ritualistic activities, such as body rocking, teeth grinding, lining up objects and resisting change with 'preservation of sameness' within their environment. Other abnormalities include uncontrolled development of imagination, marked feeding problems, peculiar sleep patterns, unpredictable fears, aggression and temper tantrums, short attention span, lack of initiative and abnormal motor movements such as tip toe walking and unusual hand movements and postures. Occasionally special isolated skills develop which usually involve tasks needing rote memory such as computation, recognition of music, jig-saws or words of songs.

Wing L 1970 The syndrome of early childhood autism. British Journal Hospital Medicine 4: 381–392
Wing L 1983 Clinical description, diagnosis and

differential diagnosis. In: Wing J, Wing L (eds) Handbook of Psychiatry 3 Psychoses of uncertain aetiology. Cambridge University Press, Cambridge

87 Poisoning by drugs is the major cause of parasuicide with lacerations, hangings and other methods collectively accounting for only 10%. Among the drug group 78% of people used prescribed drugs mostly tranquillisers, antidepressants and non-barbiturate hypnotics. In recent years barbiturate overdoses have become less common, which probably reflects changes in prescribing habits. While all types of drugs are used at all ages, non-prescribed analgesics are more commonly used by adolescents, while sedatives are more frequently taken by the older age groups. Over 50% of parasuicides seen in hospitals involve more than one drug. Self laceration, mostly involving superficial incisions on the wrists, account for 6% and injuries with firearms and explosives, hanging, suffocation, immersion and jumping together account for a very small proportion of cases. Alcohol misuse in the form of chronic problem drinking is seen in 24% of males and 7% of females who deliberately harm themselves. 50% of men and 25% of females who harm themselves have had recent intake of alcohol prior to the self-harm act.

Morgan H 1982 Deliberate self-harm. In: Granville–Grossman K (ed) Recent Advances in Clinical Psychiatry 4. Churchill Livingstone, Edinburgh

88 Brown showed that high expressed emotion predicted relapse, particularly in those patients who were in close contact with their relatives. Vaughan and Leff claimed that high expressed emotion in and close contact with relatives was causally related to relapse. Among patients spending more than thirty-five hours per week with relatives showing high expressed emotion the relapse rate was 92% for those not taking antipsychotic medication and 53% for those taking medication. Regular medication and reduced contact with relatives were protective factors. Leff attempted to reduce expressed emotion in relatives in high contact with patients by various social interventions. He showed that the effectiveness of these interventions in reducing the relapse rate extended over a two-year period. His study

showed that the relapse rate of control patients in high expressed emotion homes who took regular medication was 78% over two years, and for those patients in the trial social intervention reduced this figure to 20%. On this basis they argued that a causal role in precipitating relapse had been established for expressed emotion in relatives and a major determinant of outcome had been identified. Criticisms of this work refers to the small number of patients and in only three cases was relapse sufficient to require hospitalisation. Other previous studies showed less impressive findings but were consistent with the causal hypothesis. Recently Crow's group does not seem to support the postulated causal connection between expressed emotion and relapse in schizophrenia.

Leff J 1985 Family treatment of schizophrenia. In: Granville–Grossman K (ed) Recent Advances in Clinical Psychiatry. Churchill Livingstone, Edinburgh

McMillan J, Gold A, Crow T, Johnson A L, Johnstone E C 1986 Emotion and Relapse. British Journal of Psychiatry 148: 133–143

89 Emil Durkheim proposed a relationship between suicide and social conditions and described a number of varieties of suicide. Egoistic suicide referred to people who had been separated from the social group and hence lost their sense of integration in the community. Anomic suicide occurred in individuals who had no normative values to help them during stressful periods. Rarer types include the altruistic and fatalistic forms. Altruistic types refers to individuals who sacrifice their lives for the good of the social group and fatalistic types occurs under excessive regulation such as might occur in prison. Durkheim also found higher suicide rates in older adults, males, Protestants as compared to Catholics and Jews, the unmarried and divorced, in the upper classes, and in soldiers compared with civilians. His sociological viewpoint is still considered meaningful in western cultures.

Roy A 1986 Self-destructive behaviour. In: Hill P, Murray R, Thorley A (eds) Essentials of Postgraduate Psychiatry 2nd edn. Grune and Stratton, London

Watts C 1982 Suicide and parasuicide. In: Paykel E S (ed) Handbook of Affective Disorders. Churchill Livingstone, Edinburgh

90 Profound memory impairment of organic origin will usually be accompanied by impairment of consciousness or disruption of other cognitive functions. In psychogenic amnesia, where the subject may complain of loss of personal identity or an inability to recall lengthy periods of life, the other cognitive functions are intact and inconsistencies may be noted between the limited ability to actively recall an event on request and the subject's behaviour, which would reflect a knowledge of the same event. For example, not being able to recall the death of a relative, but behaving in a manner consistent with the fact that the deceased relative no longer existed. Other features of psychogenic amnesia are that the recall difficulty frequently centres on themes which are emotionally significant, there is often profound difficulty with recall, but the patient is able to retain new information in a normal manner or alternatively they are unable to retain any details even momentarily. In some instances psychogenic and organic amnesia occur together and it is then often impossible to distinguish the relative importance of either causative factor.

Lishman W A 1978 Symptoms and syndromes with regional affiliations. In: Organic Psychiatry. Blackwell, Oxford

Thorley A 1986 Neurosis and Personality Disorder. In: Hill P, Murray R, Thorley A (eds) Essentials of Postgraduate Psychiatry 2nd edn. Grune and Stratton, London

91 Review of the literature indicates that the prevalence rates for neuroses varies from 1–10% with a mean of 5% and that there is a marked preponderance of females. This group contains both early and late onset neuroses and all varieties of neurotic symptomatology are seen in long standing cases though they tend to have a higher degree of hypochondriacal preoccupation despite good physical health. Patients with late onset neuroses generally exhibit anxiety or depressive symptoms with depression predominating and they tend to have major physical disabilities and show a higher mortality rate than those with early onset neurosis. The prevalence of personality disorder varies from 3% to 15% with a mean of 6%.

Kay D, Bergmann K 1980 Epidemiology of mental disorder among the aged in the community. In: Birren J, Sloane R (eds) Handbook of Mental Health and Aging. Prentice-Hall, New York

92 It provides the dual function of assessment of the degree and distribution of brain atrophy and it demonstrates some potentially reversible dementias such as subdural haematomas or resectable tumours. Where doubt exists about the diagnosis, computerised tomography can be helpful but one should not rely exclusively on radiological findings. This is especially so in presenile dementia where studies have shown that the radiological diagnosis may not be sustained over time. In most patients with Alzheimer's disease scanning demonstrates sulcal widening and ventricular enlargement and while an association exists between clinical diagnosis and radiological atrophy, dementia may occur without significant changes. Studies have shown that misclassification between dementia, normal subjects and patients with affective disorder occurs in 18 to 40% of cases. An agreement of only 40% was found in one study where clinical features and CT appearance were to differentiate between Alzheimer's disease and multi-infarct dementia. New techniques of measurement of radio-attenuation density may prove of greater assistance in diagnoses since it evaluates brain substance rather than CSF space. So far CT remains an adjunct in assessment and differential diagnosis of dementia to be used along with psychometry, clinical examination, EEG, laboratory diagnoses and neurological findings.

Jacoby R, Levy R 1980 Computed Tomography in the Elderly: senior dimentias—diagnosis and functional impairment. British Journal of Psychiatry 136: 256–269

Jacoby R, Levy R, Dawson J M 1980 Computer Tomography in the Elderly 1: the normal population. British Journal of Psychiatry 136: 249–255

Bondareff W, Baldy R, Levy R 1981 Qualitative computed tomography in senile dimentias. Archives of General Psychiatry 38: 1365–1368

93 The assessment should focus mainly on the thoughts and emotions that the patient was experiencing at the time of the intent. The interview with the patient should concentrate on why it happened, what precipitated the attempt and whether he intended to die, effect a change in others behaviour or simply ensure a few hours sleep. How the patient now feels about the attempt and his future and how intensely his mood is disturbed needs to be assessed. The effect

of what you say and whether they can respond positively to assurances about their future needs careful observation. On the objective side, the seriousness of the attempted suicide needs to be assessed in terms of the method used, degree of planning, the medical consequences of the attempt and what was the probability of being rescued. Note must also be taken of any demographic features associated with an increased suicidal risk: being over 45 years, male, white, married, living alone, unemployed, in poor physical health, having alcoholism, a history of previous attempts, or a family history of suicide. Finally, the degree of support the patient has from family and friends and what the long term prognosis is for the underlying psychiatric disorder will have a bearing on the suicidal risk.

Roy A 1986 Self-destructive behaviour. In: Hill P, Murray R, Thorley A (eds) Essentials of Postgraduate Psychiatry 2nd edn. Grune and Stratton, London

94 Electroencephalography is still a useful tool in helping to distinguish functional from non-functional disorders, but because it produces a high rate of both false positive and negative findings it has a limited diagnostic role. Recordings show considerable variation between normal subjects due to constitutional factors and within individuals with changes in level of arousal, blood sugar concentration, acid-base balance and age. Furthermore, recordings are frequently sensitive to medications. In addition, mental illness in general and personality disorders in particular are associated with a high rate of EEG abnormalities. The EEG does, however, help to refute or support a clinical suspicion of an organic disorder, helps both to localise and indicate the nature of the pathology and provides useful confirmatory information in the diagnosis of epilepsy. Where there is an abnormal recording it is not very specific diagnostically, except in the case of space occupying lesions and in identifying the origin and type of epilepsy.

Cutting J, McClelland R 1986 Psychiatric manifestations of organic illness. In: Hill P, Murray R, Thorley A (eds) Essentials of Postgraduate Psychiatry 2nd edn. Grune and Stratton, London
Kiloh L G, McComas A J, Osselton J W 1972 The value and limitations of electroencephalography. In: Clinical Encephalography 3rd edn. Butterworths, London

95 The spinal fluid must be examined in every
patient with syphilis or suspected neurosyphilis as
it is the only means of detecting involvement of
the central nervous system in the asymptomatic
stage of the infection or when blood serology is
negative. In most cases of symptomatic neurosyphilis the cerebrospinal fluid shows a moderate
lymphocytosis and the protein concentration is
elevated. The Venereal Disease Research Laboratory test is positive in about 75% of cases while
the Fluorescent Treponemal Antibody-Absorption
tests and the Treponemal Pallidum Immobiliz-
ation test (TPI) are almost always positive. Possible
false positive reagin tests, due to autoimmune and
collagen diseases, can be confidently excluded
when the more specific TPI test is positive. If the
spinal fluid serology is positive but the cell count
and protein concentration are normal, increased
spinal lgG and lgM immunoglobulins concentrations and the presence of plasma cells suggest
active neurosyphilis. The colloidal gold curve is
now thought to have little diagnostic significance.

Greenwood R 1980 Neurosyphilis. Medicine
  32: 1660–1663

96 According to Russell's criteria anorexia nervosa is
characterised by specific endocrine features of
amenorrhoea in the female and decreased libido
and potency in the male, a psychopathological
disturbance characterist by a morbid fear of
becoming fat and behaviour on the patient's part
that leads to a marked loss of body weight. The
most common method of weight loss is extreme
restriction of food intake but weight loss may be
aggravated by self-induced vomiting, purging or
excessive exercise. The DSM III criteria charac-
terises anorexia nervosa as a weight loss of 25%
of original body weight, an intense fear of
becoming obese, disturbance of body image,
refusal to maintain normal body weight and an
absence of physical illness to account for the
weight loss. This diagnostic scheme is essentially
an amalgamation of Bruch's criteria which are
psychological ones such as body image disturbance, a paralysing sense of ineffectiveness and a
decreased sense of internal awareness, and
Feighner's criteria which are essentially a checklist
of symptoms. The DSM III is criticised for its
exclusion of amenorrhoea as a diagnostic criteria,
its vague definition of 'disturbed body image' and

its strict weight loss criteria of 25% which excludes milder cases.

Diagnostic and Statistical Manual of Mental Disorders 1980 3rd edn. American Psychiatric Association Washington

Russell G 1983 Anorexia nervosa and bulimia nervosa. In: Russell G, Hersov L (eds) Handbook of Psychiatry 4 The neuroses and personality disorders. Cambridge University Press, Cambridge

97 Piaget described a universally present sequence of qualitatively different cognitive models characterising the stage of personality development. He claimed that a variety of abilities appear more or less simultaneously at each stage of development because they are all generated by the same recently developed cognitive structure. The sensori-motor stage from birth to two years principally concerns the development of object permanence. The child differentiates himself from others and builds inner representations of himself and permanent outer objects. In the pre-operational stage, from two to seven years, the child shows the beginnings of symbolic play. There are four main characteristics of this stage: egocentrism, animism, pre-causal logic and authoritarian' morality. In the concrete operational stage from age seven to twelve years children lose their egocentrism, their animism and authoritarianism. The child masters conservation concepts, begins to perform logical manipulations and engage in co-operative activities with others. In the final formal operational stage the adolescent becomes capable of abstract thinking. He tries out hypotheses systematically and becomes concerned with philosophical and ideological problems. Piaget stresses the interaction of each stage of the cognitive and emotional processes.

Atkinson R, Atkinson R, Hilgard E 1983 (eds) Introduction to Psychology 8th edn. International Edition. Harcourt Brace Jovanovich, New York

Piaget J, Inhelder B 1969 The psychology of the child. Routledge & Kegan Paul, London

98 Organic impairment may be indicated by a significant discrepancy between verbal and performance scores on the Wechsler Adult Intelligence Scale. A discrepancy between these tests and a low performance score can aid the discrimination between dementia and functional disorders, but they are not very satisfactory. The Wechsler Memory Scale is

widely used to detect minor degrees of diffuse brain damage and to clarify the extent to which memory functions are impaired out of proportion to other cognitive factors. Kendrick and his colleagues claim that a consolidation of the synonym learning test with a motor test designed to measure the speed of copying digits yielded a diagnostic discrimination accuracy of over 90%. The synonym learning test which is based on the Mill Hill Vocabulary Scale involves the learning of definitions of unfamiliar words. Also of help in discriminating these two conditions is the paired associate learning test elaborated by Inglis. This test which is designed to be sensitive to memory impairment, involves the repetition of a previously learned paired word when the stimulus word is given. Neuropsychological assessments may demonstrate focal abnormalities of higher cortical function which would strongly indicate an organic illness. These would include tests of orientation, spatial perception, block and stick construction tasks and tests for dysphasic errors.

Kendrick D C, Gibson A J, Moyes I C A 1979 The revised Kendrick Battery: Clinical studies. British Journal of Social and Clinical Psychology 18 (3): 329–340

Miller E 1980 Cognitive assessment of the older adult. In: Birren J, Sloane B (eds) Handbook of Mental Health and Aging. Prentice-Hall, New York

99   This is an observer rating scale for depressive disorders. It was one of the first designed and is now widely used in drug trials and as a measure of the reliability of other rating instruments. It consists of 17 items covering the most common symptoms of all types of depression and many of the items are concerned with somatic symptoms. It has a high inter-rater reliability and correlates well with global clinical ratings of depression. The scale can be completed in the course of ordinary clinical interviews, although it is always advisable to obtain supplementary information. The structure of the scale makes it score highly when somatic symptoms are present, but it tends to underestimate the severity of the depression when those symptoms are few or absent. Another disadvantage is that it cannot be used frequently as it is intended to record the patient's condition for the preceding week or two.

Hamilton M 1976 The role of rating scales in psychiatry. Psychological medicine 6: 347–349

100   This is an invaluable tool in psychiatry in that it can detect intracranial lesions and so help distinguish functional from organic disorders, without being invasive or exposing the patient to large doses of radiation. It can locate areas of localised cerebral oedema, tumours, abscesses, haematomas and help distinguish between infarction and haemorrhage. It is particularly useful in detecting cortical atrophy and ideally any patient with dementing features should have a CAT scan so that unsuspected lesions such as a tumour or subdural haematoma are not overlooked. In addition it can help to distinguish dementia from pseudo-dementia. However, there are limitations to its use: radiological 'atrophy' can be detected without dementias in healthy subjects and dementia of the Alzheimer's type can occur without 'atrophy' in some 15% of instances respectively. Small or very early diffuse lesions can be missed, especially those at the base of the skull or near the anterior intracranial optic pathways. Subdural haematomas which are isodense with brain tissue will not be detected. Features of cortical atrophy have been found on CAT scans of patients with alcoholism, schizophrenia and psychotic depression, but the place for this radiological technique has not been established in the clinical management of these disorders.

Cutting J, McClelland R 1986 Psychiatric manifestations of organic illness. In: Hill P, Murray R, Thorley A (eds) Essentials of Postgraduate Psychiatry 3rd edn. Grune and Stratton, London
Jacoby R J, Levy R 1980 Computerised tomography in the elderly: Affective disorder. British Journal of Psychiatry 136: 270–275

101   The team should provide the full range of services and continuing emotional support over a long period of time. From the initial discovery of the handicap, parents need help to cope with their grief and adjust their expectations of the child. The multidisciplinary team provides early and factual information about the extent of handicap and its prognosis for the family and involves the family in the assessment of the handicap. Counselling as soon as the diagnosis is made may identify vulnerable families and help them meet the demands of the situation. Where inherited conditions are involved genetic counselling should be available. Over the years parents will need continuing emotional support and advice to help them

achieve a balance between the needs of the retarded child and those of the rest of the family. They also need practical information on how to teach basic daily living skills and manage behaviour problems. Teaching kits, of which Portage is one example, and parents' workshops have the advantage of involving parents in a mutual support system. Families may be helped by periods of respite from the burden of care by providing babysitting arrangements, short term residential care while on holiday or help from foster families. The social worker may arrange for dental care, financial allowances, grants, the provision of aids and special educational provisions. Future plans for possible residential care and long term prognosis must be discussed with the family to allay anxiety as they get older. Voluntary society membership should be encouraged as these bodies provide useful support for the family and fulfil an important complementary role alongside the professional services.

Shearer M, Shearer D 1972 The portage project: A model for early childhood education. Exceptional Child 39: 210–217

Taylor E, Bicknell J 1986 The psychiatry of mental handicap. In: Hill P, Murray R, Thorley A (eds) Essentials of Postgraduate Psychiatry 2nd edn. Grune and Stratton, London

102 Prevention of mild handicap, because of its numerous and less discrete causes is very difficult. Improvement in the socio-economic factors such as housing, employment, nutrition, education of parents and children and health services would often help prevention. More specifically, prevention largely depends on genetic counselling, early detection of foetal abnormalities during pregnancy and safe delivery. Amniocentesis, fetoscopy and ultrasound scanning can reveal chromosomal abnormalities and some inborn errors of metabolism. Regular antenatal attendance, dietetic counselling, identification of high risk mothers, cautious use of drugs, early diagnosis and treatment of maternal infections, reduced intake of alcohol and cessation of smoking may all reduce the prevalence of handicap. Atraumatic delivery with good paediatric liaison is also an essential aspect of prevention. Improved neonatal care for premature and low birth weight infants can prevent retardation but may also bring about survival in some retarded children who would

otherwise have died. Screening for hypothyroidism, phenylketonuria and other inborn errors
of metabolism is very important. In the post-natal
period adequate nutrition, prevention and early
treatment of infections and prevention of accidents may reduce the prevalence of handicap.

Nelson Textbook of Paediatrics 1983 (eds) Vaughan V,
    McKay R, Behrmann R 12th edn. Saunders,
    London

103   Attempts to apply behavioural and analytical
psychotherapeutic techniques to reverse gender
identity in transsexuals have largely failed though
there are some reports of undecided transsexuals
being helped by behavioural approaches. Most
patients relentlessly pursue sex reassignment
operations. In practice the two year 'real-life test',
which means that the patient lives fully in the
chosen life before irreversible surgery is contem-
plated, should be applied. If the patient copes well
with this test and resolves the social and personal
difficulties of changing gender role, then surgery
is likely to be followed with good adjustment.
This relatively long period before surgery is
important as the transsexual urges may vary in
intensity or may depend on situational factors
such as the views of the current sexual partner.
Before reconstructive surgery is undertaken, male
patients are generally given oestrogen to reduce
libido and this also may produce some breast
development and soften body hair; female patients
are given testosterone to induce hair growth,
suppress menstruation and deepen the voice.
Facial electrolysis, voice and social skills training
may help to increase the authenticity of gender
role behaviour. After surgical reconstruction
counselling should continue to help adjustment to
the new role.

Bancroft J 1983 Human sexuality and its
    problems. Churchill Livingstone, Edinburgh
Money J, Ambinder R 1978 Two year, real life
    diagnostic test: Rehabilitation versus cure. In:
    Bradly J, Brodie H K H (eds) Controversy in
    Psychiatry. Saunders, Philadelphia

104   Perceptual abnormalities can affect all sensory
modalities in schizophrenia. Auditory hallucinations are the most common while visual, olfactory,
gustatory and tactile hallucinations are uncommon
in the absence of hallucinatory voices. Elementary

hallucinations are not so prominent but patients may hear buzzing, whistling and other noises which are often attributed to the machinations of the persecutors. The hallucinatory voices in schizophrenia vary considerably in duration, content, clarity and in the effect they have on the patient's thoughts, behaviour and emotions. Schneider held that specific types of auditory hallucinations are characteristic of schizophrenia. These specific types include: voices repeating the subject's thoughts aloud, two or more voices discussing the subject with reference to him in the third person and a running commentary on the subject's thoughts or behaviour. Visual hallucinations are rare in schizophrenia and throw doubt on the diagnosis. Bodily hallucinations are quite common so that the patient may complain of sensations of heat, cold, pain, or electric shocks. Hallucinations of smell may occur as do hallucinations of taste.

Hamilton M (ed) 1974 Fish's clinical psychopathology. Wright, Bristol
Kendell R E 1988 Schizophrenia. In: Kendell R E, Zealley A K (eds) Companion to Psychiatric Studies, 4th edn. Churchill Livingstone, Edinburgh

105 Withdrawal symptoms usually begin within 4–12 hours, peak at 24–48 hours and gradually subside over 7–10 days. However, the timing of this abstinence syndrome and its duration varies with the different opiates, duration of dependence and with the dose on which the patient was dependent. Physical effects are mainly due to sympathetic and parasympathetic overactivity. Prominent symptoms include craving for drugs, yawning, lacrimation, dilated pupils, tachycardia, marked agitation and irritability and gastrointestinal symptoms such as nausea, vomiting, diarrhoea and abdominal cramps. A subjective feeling of coldness occurs accompanied by pilo-erection, increased perspiration and flushing of the face and neck. Rhinorrhoea develops with paroxysms of sneezing. Sleep disturbance due to an increase in REM sleep may last for up to two months. Psychological and cognitive elements of dependence may persist for some time after the physical effects of withdrawal have receded.

Hamid Ghodse A 1983 Drug dependence and intoxication. In: Lader M (ed) Handbook of Psychiatry 2. Mental disorders and somatic illness. Cambridge University Press, Cambridge

106   This is a descriptive term covering a wide range of bizarre behaviour and persistent accusations in which there is a common theme of preoccupation with the sexual partner's infidelity. The sexual partner is constantly interrogated, denial not being accepted and attempts to prove this infidelity are constantly being made. Such behaviour leads to frequent quarrelling, bitterness and sometimes to violence. Between one-third to one-half of patients have a psychotic disorder of a paranoid or depressive type. Neuroses and personality disorders account for one-third to one-half of patients. A variety of personality disorders, chiefly paranoid personalities as well as asthenic and sociopathic types have been described. Alcoholism as a primary diagnoses accounts for less than 7% of the total. Drug addictions such as those of amphetamine and cocaine, cerebral organic states, endocrinopathies, lead poisoning, epilepsy, Parkinson's disease, dementia, Huntington's chorea and the punch drunk syndrome are also associated with morbid jealousy.

Cobb J 1979 Morbid jealousy. British Journal of Hospital Medicine May 511–518.

Shepherd M 1961 Morbid jealousy: Some clinical and social aspects of a psychiatric syndrome. Journal of Mental Science 107: 657

107   These are delusions that are in keeping with and understandable in the context of the patient's mood. A depressed patient will usually think in a negative manner and as the depression intensifies the negative thoughts can develop into delusions. For example, the patient might initially be concerned about his finances and this concern can gradually develop into a conviction that he is bankrupt. The content of depressive delusions usually centre on money, religion, good and evil and health. Likewise the delusions of mania are usually understandable in the context of the patient's mood and their content relates to the patient's over-estimation of his abilities in a wide variety of situations.

Hamilton M 1985 Classification of psychiatric disorders. In: Fish's Clinical Psychopathology 2nd edn. Wright, Bristol

Tyrer S, Shopsin B 1982 Symptoms and assessment of mania. In: Handbook of Affective Disorders (ed) Paykel E S Churchill Livingstone, Edinburgh

108　The assessment should be 'action orientated' as its purpose is the definition of the patient's problem in a way which will suggest specific behaviours for modification and specific treatment procedures. A detailed description of the problem must be sought with details concerning the psychological, cognitive, emotional and behavioural aspects of the problems. Clarification of the problem includes identifying the cues and antecedent events and the people and circumstances which maintain the problem behaviour. Other important modifying factors include medication, associated personality or psychiatric problems, physical disorders, the presence of concurrent stress factors in the patient's life, family relationships and his reactions to the problem. A motivational analysis attempts to isolate the various incentives and adverse conditions specific to the patient. An analysis of self-control provides information on the patient's capacity for participation in treatment. Analysis of the patient's social relationships and environment assesses the social resources which may help or hinder him in treatment. In addition, a full functional analysis should include some observation, self-monitoring, simulated and unobtrusive measurement. Other rating scales such as the self-rating scale for anxiety and the fear survey schedule may help provide a global assessment of symptoms. The behavioural analysis is discussed with the patient and by the end of the assessment, agreement for the proposed programme of treatment should be concluded with him.

Kaufer F H, Saslow G 1969 Behavioural diagnosis. In: Frank C H (ed) Behaviour Therapy: Appraisal and Status. McGraw-Hill, New York
Peck D F, McGuire R J 1988 Behavioural approaches in psychiatry. In: Kendell R E, Zealley A K (eds) Companion to Psychiatric Studies, 4th edn. Churchill Livingstone, Edinburgh

109　Approximately 10–20% of persons who exhibit deliberate self harm behaviour commit suicide in the year after the episode and the long term suicide risk rises to 10%. The risk of suicide increases in the older age group particularly among males. Other correlates include: many previous attempts, a serious attempt, social isolation, unemployment or retirement, widowed or divorced, poor physical health and a suicide note. A subgroup with severe personality disorders and interpersonal conflicts and who are often alcohol or drug dependent may commit suicide while acutely depressed.

Dorpat T, Ripley H 1967 The relationship between attempted suicide and committed suicide. Comprehensive Psychiatry 8: 74–79

Kreitman N 1977 (ed.) Parasuicide. Wiley, Chichester

110   This term, coined by Morselli in 1886, describes a condition where the individual persistently complains about some presumed defect in physical appearance which he or she is convinced is very noticeable to others, although in reality the appearance is within normal limits. The most common sites of complaint are the nose, ears, mouth, breasts and penis, but any part of the body may be the focus. One of the difficulties in the use of this term is that some authors regard it as a discrete psychiatric illness while others see dysmorphophobia as a symptom of an underlying disorder. The typical picture of the discrete illness is of a young individual with narcissistic, obsessional or schizoid personality traits who believes that his or her perceived ugliness is noticeable to others. This belief is an over-valued idea. Dysmorphophobia may be either an over-valued idea or a delusion and present in a wide range of psychiatric disorders. These disorders include schizophrenia, affective illness, personality disorder, psychotic states or severe neuroses. The treatment is usually that which is appropriate for the underlying condition. Phenothiazines can be useful if the symptom is delusional. Cosmetic surgery might be indicated if mild deformity is present, although the patient may have unrealistic expectations. Some patients are helped by supportive psychotherapy, but many are resistant to change.

Hay G G 1970 Psychiatric aspects of cosmetic nasal operations. British Journal of Psychiatry 116: 85–97

Hay G G 1970 Dysmorphophobia. British Journal of Psychiatry 116: 399–406

Thomas C S 1984 Dysmorphophobia: A question of definition. British Journal of Psychiatry 144: 513–517

111   Homosexual men either seek help for sexual dysfunction affecting their homosexual relationship or because they desire to change their orientation. The methods used in treating the

functional difficulties are similar to those used in heterosexual men. Masters and Johnson treated homosexual men for dysfunctions such as premature ejaculation and impotence and their results in homosexual men were comparable to those obtained in heterosexual men. Psychoanalytical and behavioural approaches are used in treatment of homosexual sexual conversion. The evidence for change with psychoanalysis remains equivocal and treatment is very lengthy. Behavioural techniques include aversive therapy, to decrease the deviant interest and a variety of approaches to increase heterosexual interest such as orgasmic reconditioning, fading, shaping, biofeedback and aversive relief. Masters and Johnson tend to treat homosexuals with a partner of the opposite sex. While their results are favourable, they have a highly selected population. Educative, psychotherapeutic and social skills approaches are employed to help the homosexual adjust to his sexual orientation.

Bancroft J 1983 Human sexuality and its problems. Churchill Livingstone, Edinburgh

Masters W, Johnson V 1979 Homosexuality in perspective. Little Brown, Boston

112 Two groups of elderly alcoholics have been identified: those who have life long histories of habitual heavy drinking accounting for two-thirds of the total group and those who turn to alcohol in excess in old age. Those alcoholics from the first group tend to have symptoms of the alcohol dependence syndrome and have personality traits similar to those of younger alcoholics. The whole range of psychiatric and organic disorder secondary to alcohol are noted in this group. Late onset alcoholics tend to have more stable personalities and good work records. They are rarely physically dependent on alcohol, the problems being essentially those of alcohol related falls, confusion and self-neglect. The change from abstinence or social drinking to problem drinking can be dated to the not too distant past usually following changes in life circumstances, particularly losses. Bereavement, retirement and physical disability have been identified as major precipitants of this condition. Reported prevalence rates for alcoholism range from 0% to 16% for males and from 0% to 0.6% for females. Brody estimated the prevalence at less than 3% in those over sixty-five years, but noted that up to 15% of

elderly people seen medically have alcohol related disorders, such as confusion or alcoholic dementia.

Brody J A 1982 Aging and alcohol abuse. Journal of American Geriatrics Society 30 (2): 123–126

Rosin A J, Glatt M M 1971 Alcohol excess in the elderly. Quarterly Journal of Studies in Alcoholism 32: 53–59

113 Management is based on a comprehensive assessment of the developmental and bowel training histories, family dynamics and social stresses and on an evaluation of possible organic factors so that the type of faecal soiling can be identified. Abdominal and rectal examination will usually identify any local pathology but occasionally X-ray and further studies may be needed as in the case of Hirschsprung's disease. Treatment of constipation with overflow incontinence starts with enemas and proceeds rapidly to maintenance bulk forming agents or laxatives. A bowel training routine using star charts and rewards is often successful as the sole treatment. Involvement of the parents in the retraining programme is advantageous. Other behavioural methods have been used such as the direct teaching of correct defaecation with modelling, relaxation and biofeedback techniques. Retraining approaches are nearly always combined with individual psychotherapy and parental counselling. Family therapy can be a useful adjunct along with behavioural modification. For the more difficult problems in-patient facilities may be required.

Taylor E 1983 Disturbances of toilet function. In: Russell G, Hersov L (eds) Handbook of Psychiatry 4. The neuroses and personality disorders. Cambridge University Press, Cambridge

114 The term was coined to describe the emotional impact that relatives had on patients and it was used first in reference to schizophrenics. Brown found that high expressed emotion predicted relapse in schizophrenia, particularly in those patients in close contact with their relatives and Vaughan and Leff claimed that high 'expressed emotion' and close contact with relatives were causally related to schizophrenia. Studies have shown that over 50% relapse over a nine-month period in high expressed emotion homes compared to 13% in low expressed emotion homes and that medication and low contact with relatives are

protective factors. The assessment of expressed emotion is derived from the Camberwell Family Interview, which has four main components: critical comments, over-involvement, hostility and warmth, of which the first two are regarded as the crucial measures. Expressed emotion has been measured in various cultural settings and in a variety of diagnostic groups. The relationship between expressed emotion and outcome of schizophrenia holds good across cultural and linguistic divides. Expressed emotion has also been linked with the relatives of depressed patients, anorexic and obese patients.

Kendell R E 1988 Schizophrenia. In: Kendell R E, Zealley A K (eds) Companion to Psychiatric Studies, 4th edn. Churchill Livingstone, Edinburgh

Leff J 1985 Family treatment of schizophrenia. In: Granville–Grossman K (ed) Recent Advances in Clinical Psychiatry, 5. Churchill Livingstone, Edinburgh

115 This disorder is generally considered to be an attenuated form of schizophrenia, occurring late in life and it is characterised by prominent paranoid delusions with or without hallucinations. The central feature is a well systematised paranoid delusional state but occasionally some patients present with Schneiderian first rank symptoms. It occurs predominantly in elderly females who are socially isolated, some 40% show longstanding deafness and a minority are also visually impaired. The onset is insidious. Their premorbid personality is often described as egocentric, jealous, opinionated, suspicious or shy and reserved. A high proportion are single or divorced and many have difficulties in maintaining relationships. Despite a chronic course affective, volitional and intellectual aspects of the personality remain fairly well preserved.

Graham P 1982 Late paraphrenia. British Journal Hospital Medicine 27(5): 522–530

Post F 1982 Functional disorders. In: Levy R, Post F (eds) The Psychiatry of Late Life. Blackwell, Oxford

116 Once the medical consequences of the overdose have been dealt with the risk of another suicide attempt should be assessed. If the patient's subjective account of the episode, the objective facts such as the method used and the probability of being rescued or the presence of demographic

features associated with an increased risk of suicide indicate a high risk of further serious suicidal attempts, then adequate preventative steps should be taken until the motivation for the suicidal behaviour is no longer present. If there is a supportive family member available and the patient has not needed admission for medical management of the overdose then it is often appropriate that the patient be treated on an outpatient basis. When medical admission has been necessary it is essential to ensure that there is adequate support at home and that a responsible relative is able to take control before the patient is discharged. If these facilities are not available or if the underlying depression is very profound admission to hospital for psychiatric treatment should be recommended.

Hillard J R 1983 Emergency management of the suicidal patient. In: Walker J I (ed) Psychiatric Emergencies. Lippincott, Philadelphia

Urbaitis J C 1983 Suicide attempts and risks. In: Psychiatric Emergencies. Appleton-Century-Crofts, Norwalk, Connecticut

117 The central characteristic is that clothes appropriate to the opposite sex assume a fetishistic quality and cross-dressing is associated with sexual arousal and orgasm. The term transvestite is generally confined to those who have fetishistic transvestism, though transvestism may occur in a number of different conditions such as severe psychotic illness, in association with homosexuality, or temporal lobe disorder, or as a transient phenomenon in normal adolescence. Transvestites may become excited by a simple female garment and wear it intermittently to produce sexual arousal before masturbation. Others have a desire to be completely cross-dressed and this is associated with genital excitement and sexual gratification. Others completely cross-dress and learn to live as women. Typically such a transvestite wants to pass as a woman while cross-dressed but does not want to be a woman. Occasionally transsexualism may develop where the transvestite wants to be a woman. Transvestites are almost always male, most are married and they prefer female sexual partners and will generally try to keep their cross-dressing secret. The cross-dressing usually starts in adolescence.

Bancroft J 1983 Human sexuality and its problems. Churchill Livingstone, Edinburgh

Wakeling A 1983 Transvestism, transsexualism and
exhibitionism. In: Russell G, Hersov L (eds)
Handbook of Psychiatry 4 The neuroses and
personality disorders. Cambridge University Press,
Cambridge

118 This refers to memory loss for events prior to the
injury or lesion and is measured from the time of
the last clear memory. Usually it lasts only from
a few seconds to a minute and the subject is
unable to recall any details of the period. Estimates of its duration should only be made after
the subject has recovered from any post-traumatic
amnesia. Retrograde amnesia is thought to result
from information which has registered just before
the injury, but has not had time to be consolidated
as a memory. The duration of the amnesia is not
as reliable a guide of the severity of the injury as
that of post-traumatic amnesia. Retrograde
amnesia, lasting days or weeks, may occasionally
be seen with severe head injury or organic disease,
but its exact mechanism is unclear and psychogenic factors may be important.

Lishman W A 1978 Head Injury. In: Organic
Psychiatry. Blackwell, Oxford

119 Personality traits which have emerged from
various studies include poor impulse control, a
need for immediate gratification, poor self-esteem,
poor socialisation, hostility and self-destructive
tendencies. Employing the Minnesota Multiphasic
Personality Inventory, over 95% have abnormal
profiles, mostly on the psychopathic scales, with
little contribution coming from neurotic or
psychotic profiles. Addicts score higher on 'sensation seeking' scales. Heroin users reveal more
aggression and sociopathic characteristics while
alcoholics show more depressive, anxiety and
neurotic traits. Pure heroin users appear to be
better adjusted psychologically than polydrug
abusers. Overall, while personality factors may
contribute to drug abuse, there is no evidence of
a specific personality type which invariably leads
to addiction.

Gersick K E, Grady K, Sexton E, Lyons M 1981
Personality and Sociodemographic factors in
adolescent drug use. NIDA Research Monograph
38: 39–56
Gordon A M 1985 Psychological aspects of drug
abuse. In: Granville–Grossman K (ed) Recent
Advances in Clinical Psychiatry 5. Churchill
Livingstone, Edinburgh

120 Evidence from twin and adoption studies seem to indicate that genetic factors contribute a liability towards alcoholism. The prevalence of alcoholism among the parents and siblings of alcoholics is about two-to-three times that of the general population and the morbidity risk of alcoholism for an individual with one alcoholic parent is 25%. Kaij showed a concordance rate for monozygotic twins of 70% compared to 32% for dizygotic twins. Replication of these studies show less striking results. Goodwin reported in his adoptive studies that the sons of alcoholics were four times more likely to develop alcoholism than adoptees without alcoholic biological parents. They also compared the adopted-away sons of alcoholics with their brothers who were raised by the alcoholic parent and found similar rates of alcoholism. These controversial findings have been supported by two other adoptive studies. The genetic contribution may determine personality traits, psychiatric disorders or an as yet unidentified biochemical disorder which predisposes to alcoholism. The existence of at least two genetically different types of susceptibility to alcoholism has been postulated; in one type, adult onset alcohol abuse with minimal criminality may be present in either parent and alcohol dependence is expressed in both sons and daughters, while in the other form the mode of inheritance seems to be patrilinear, hence the males have an adolescent onset of alcoholism and criminal behaviour.

Gurling H, Murray R, Clifford C 1981 Investigations into the genetics of alcohol dependence and into its effects on brain function. In: Gedda L, Parisi P, Nance W (eds) Twin Research 3 C 77–87. Alan Liss, New York

Murray R 1986 Alcoholism. In: Hill P, Murray R, Thorley A (eds) Essentials of Postgraduate Psychiatry 2nd edn. Grune and Stratton, London

121 There are many different forms of post head injury syndromes and they can be best grouped as follows: cognitive impairment, personality changes, neuroses and psychoses and the post-concussional syndrome. In Hillbom's follow-up study of war time penetrating head injuries, he found that 2% had cognitive impairment, 18% had personality changes, 8% had a psychotic disorder and some 11% had a severe neurosis. Comparable figures have emerged from studies of non-penetrating head injuries and follow up studies have

shown that some two-thirds have psychiatric sequelae six years later. The post-concussional syndrome occurs in the majority of those with head injuries and about 50% have symptoms at six weeks.

Cutting J, McClelland R 1986 Psychiatric manifestations of organic illness. In: Hill P, Murray R, Thorley A (eds) Essentials of Postgraduate Psychiatry 2nd edn. Grune and Stratton, London
Lishman W A 1978 Head Injury. In: Organic Psychiatry. Blackwell, Oxford

122 Coma is the extreme of impairment of consciousness and while it may superficially resemble sleep it can be distinguished by its relative unresponsiveness to internal and external stimuli. A person in a deep sleep can be roused, will have corneal, tendon and plantar reflexes and will awaken in response to a distended bladder. Comatose patients will be unable to recall any dream activity as their ability to register and retain information is impaired. Finally EEG recording may be helpful in distinguishing between the two states.

Kiloh L G, McComas A J, Osselton J W 1972 Infective and Non-Infective Encephalopathies. In: Clinical Electroencephalography 3rd edn. Butterworth, London
Lishman W A 1978 Cardinal psychological features of cerebral disorder. In: Organic Psychiatry. Blackwell, Oxford

123 A previous act of deliberate self harm is one of the highest predictive factors emphasising the tendency for deliberate self harm behaviour to be self perpetuating. A history of previous psychiatric treatment and having a criminal record are also significant factors. Other correlates associated with repetitious self harm behaviour include drug and alcohol abuse, unemployment, membership of lower social classes, separation from spouse, loss of mother before age 15, regret at surviving the first episode, initial episodes not precipitated by any stress and a diagnosis of sociopathy. Some research workers suggest that being widowed, divorced or separated should also be a positive predictor of repetition. Approximately 20–30% of patients make further attempts at self harm within twelve months.

Buglass D, Horton J 1974 A scale for predicting subsequent suicidal behaviour. British Journal of Psychiatry 124: 573–578

Kreitman N 1988 Suicide and parasuicide. In: Kendell
R E, Zealley A K (eds) Companion to Psychiatric
Studies, 4th edn. Churchill Livingstone, Edinburgh

124 Treatment is imprecise and empirical as the aetiology is not clearly understood. One of the main
difficulties is to distinguish true depressive symptoms from social withdrawal, flattened affect, drug
induced Parkinsonism and the effects of institutionalisation in chronic patients. A common treatment is a combination of neuroleptic medication
and tricyclic antidepressants or tricyclics alone.
Prusoff studied out patient depressed schizophrenics and showed some improvement with use
of amitriptyline and perphenazine, but only after
four months of treatment. Others report that
phenothiazines are as effective alone as when
combined with amitriptyline and that the
combined treatments produce a significant increase
in side-effects. The effectiveness of lithium has
not been proved in schizophrenia but may show
good response in schizo-affective disorder. Other
non-pharmacological treatments include supportive psychotherapy, vocational rehabilitation and
family and social interventions.

Hirsch S 1982 Medication and physical treatment of
schizophrenia. In: Wing J, Wing L (eds) Handbook
of Psychiatry 3 Psychoses of uncertain aetiology.
Cambridge University Press, Cambridge
Johnson D A W 1981 (a) Studies of depressive
symptoms in schizophrenia:
  I   Prevalence of depression and its possible causes
  II   A two-year longitudinal study of symptoms.
  III A double blind trial of orphenadrine against
       placebo.
  IV   A double blind trial of nortriptyline for depression
       in chronic schizophrenia.
British Journal of Psychiatry 139: 89–101

125 Fairburn has described a cognitive approach to
treatment of bulimia nervosa. This has three
stages and incorporates establishment of a normal
regular eating habit, cessation of laxative and
diuretic abuse, education regarding the physical
side effects of binging, detailed self-monitoring of
eating habits, problem solving training and
cognitive restructuring. This approach is relatively
effective in the short term and has gained wide
acceptance but its long term efficacy is still uncertain. Cognitive approaches have been used in
anorexia nervosa and obesity but their efficacy is

very uncertain. Garner and Bemis use a cognitive therapy in anorexia nervosa which is very similar to Beck's treatment for depression, but so far its effectiveness has not been evaluated.

Fairburn C 1984 A cognitive behavioural approach for bulimia. In: Garner D M, Garfinkel P E (eds) Handbook of Psychotherapy for Anorexia Nervosa and Bulimia. Guilford Press, New York

Garner D M, Bemis K M 1982 A cognitive-behavioural approach to anorexia nervosa. Cognitive Therapy and Research 6: 123–150

126 The possibilities of disintegrative psychosis, developmental dysphasia, schizophrenia and elective mutism must be considered. Disintegrative psychosis differs from autism in that the onset is usually at a later age, there is loss of cognitive skills with marked regression of language, speech and bowel and bladder control in an otherwise normally developing child. Schizophrenia in children rarely presents before the age of seven, resembles adult schizophrenia in its psychopathology, genetics and epidemiology and even the most affected children are of normal intelligence. Elective mutism differs from autism in that the child speaks normally in some situations, shows normal social attachments and does not show autistic abnormalities in play. Developmental dysphasia may present with stereotypies and social withdrawal but non-verbal communication and imagination are normal. Landau's syndrome of acquired aphasia with convulsions is rare but may be difficult to differentiate. Affective psychosis has been identified in children and can be diagnosed on the clinical picture. Similarly, obsessional illness and phobias can be diagnosed by examining the child's whole behaviour patterns and cognitive development. Mentally handicapped children often show autistic symptomatology and differentiation can be difficult in the more severely retarded. Abnormal bonding, parental neglect and abuse and institutional rearing may present with language delay, behavioural problems and deviant social interactions. However, with these behavioural disturbances there is usually a normal social reciprocity, an absence of specific autistic speech anomalies and an improvement in cognition, speech, social and imaginative development when the child is placed in the appropriate environment. Blind and deaf children may also show features of stereotyped behaviour and unrespon-

siveness which may resemble autism. Occasionally Asperger's syndrome may cause diagnostic difficulties.

Wing L 1982 Clinical description, diagnosis and differential diagnoses. In: Wing J, Wing L (eds) Handbook of Psychiatry 3 Psychoses of uncertain aetiology. Cambridge University Press, Cambridge

127 The most common disorder is an acute paranoid psychosis which is virtually indistinguishable from paranoid schizophrenia. The paranoid delusions occur in a setting of clear consciousness with auditory, visual or tactile hallucinations. A predominance of visual hallucinations, to an extent which is unusual in schizophrenia, and an absence of formal thought disorder are useful diagnostic clues. Stereotyped, repetitive behaviour persisting for several hours may occur after large doses of amphetamines. This stereotyped behaviour may occur as part of an amphetamine induced psychotic state or as an isolated phenomenon. Amphetamine psychosis usually follows a benign course with significant improvement occurring within days of cessation of the drug. Chronic users experience fatigue, sleepiness, hunger and depression on withdrawal. Occasionally, suicidal behaviour may be a prominent feature. Brain damage following chronic use has been postulated but it remains unconfirmed.

Connell P H 1958 Amphetamine psychoses. Maudsley Monograph 5. Chapman and Hall, London
Ritson E B, Chick J 1988 Dependence on alcohol and other drugs. In: Kendell R E, Zealley A K (eds) Companion to Psychiatric Studies, 4th edn. Churchill Livingstone, Edinburgh

128 This, which is also referred to as 'formal thought disorder', is a disturbance of conceptual or abstract thinking. Bleuler considered that the basic disorder was a disturbance of association that gave rise to changeable and unclear thinking. The associations between one phrase and the next were guided by trivial associations such as sound, alliteration or totally irrelevant connections. He believed that the incompleteness of ideas was the result of condensation, displacement and symbolism. Cameron considered over inclusiveness to be an outstanding feature while Goldstein claimed that loss of abstract thinking, resulting in concreteness, was the basic failure. Carl Schneider

considered schizophrenic language disorder to be characterised by fusion, substitution, omission and derailment. In derailment the train of thought slips into another direction; in substitution a major thought is mixed up with a subsidiary one; in fusion there is an interweaving of heterogenous elements, in omission the chain of thought is interrupted while in drivelling sequences of thought are fairly well formed and organised but are mixed up together in confusion. In schizophrenic language disorder disruption of conceptual thinking and the reduced consistency within the expression of ideas means that the words spoken are less predictable or show 'decreased redundancy' compared to that of normal language.

Fish F J 1984 Fish's Schizophrenia 3rd edn. Hamilton M (ed) Wright, Bristol
Mullen P E 1986 The mental state and states of mind. In: Hill P, Murray R, Thorley A (eds) Essentials of Postgraduate Psychiatry 2nd edn. Grune and Stratton, London

129   Yes. The proportion of 47 XXY males among male psychiatric in-patients is four to five times that in the general population. There is an increased rate of all types of mental disorder, but depression and paranoid symptoms are most common. Their personality characteristics have been described as timid, neurasthenic, with poor frustration control, decreased libido and gynaecoid features. While many with this syndrome have a normal intelligence quotient, it is significantly associated with mild mental retardation. The severity of mental retardation is associated with an increasing number of X chromosomes.

Bancroft J, Axworthy D, Ratcliffe S 1982 The personality and psychosexual development of boys with 47 XXY chromosome constitution. Journal of Child Psychology and Psychiatry 23: 169–180
Gath A 1985 Chromosomal anomalies. In: Rutter M, Hersov L (eds) Child and Adolescent Psychiatry 2nd edn. Blackwell, Oxford

130   Barton, in 1959, first drew attention to a syndrome characterised by apathy, loss of interest and initiative, lack of individuality, submissiveness and deterioration of personal habits seen among in-mates of institutions such as prisons and psychiatric hospitals. This syndrome is termed institutionalisation or institutional neuroses. Barton considered that institutionalism was largely a

product of the social structure of the institution such as lack of personal possessions, asocialisation, loss of responsibility and authoritarian and pessimistic staff attitudes. Wing and Brown in the 1970s studied patient activity in three hospitals. Poor social milieu was found to be closely related to social withdrawal, blunting of affect and poverty of speech. Improvement in patients' clinical and social responses were most highly correlated with increase in work activity and decrease in unoccupied time. They showed an improvement in about one-third of long stay patients who participated in an activity programme and who were previously affected by institutionalisation. In the 1950s and '60s institutionalism was considered a major factor in deterioration of schizophrenics in long stay hospital accommodation. However, it is now understood that their deterioration is largely a product of the illness itself and may occur in people who have never been admitted to a psychiatric hospital.

Gelder M, Gath D, Mayou R 1982 (eds) The Oxford Textbook of Psychiatry. Oxford University Press, Oxford.

Johnstone E C, Owens D G C, Gold A, Crow T S, MacMillan J F 1981 Institutionalisation and the defects of schizophrenics. British Journal of Psychiatry 139: 195–203

131 The main techniques used in social skills training are modelling, coaching, role playing, social reinforcement, shaping and modification of expectancies. The approach has a strongly educational aspect. Most often the training is done through group sessions and the participants are encouraged to meet between sessions and practice the skills and exercises to which they have been introduced. The programme initially involves assessment of the patient's difficulties and a hierarchy of targets are then arranged. A target behaviour is practised within the group using combinations of coaching, modelling and rehearsal. Patients are then encouraged, through homework assignments, to test out these exercises in real life situations and to report back to the group on the success or failure. These exercises are then analysed and the procedures repeated with new situations until the patient has a repertoire of assertive skills. During the group sessions various components of social skills are taught. These components include appropriate facial expressions, eye contact, posture, correct

vocal intonation and other varieties of self-assertion such as giving and receiving compliments and initiating and maintaining conversations. Sessions also devote time to the recognition of emotions and to the effects on others of adopting assertive and non-assertive attitudes and irrational negative beliefs.

Falloon I R H, Lindley P, McDonald R, Marks I M 1977 Social skills training of out-patient groups: A controlled study of rehearsal and homework. British Journal of Psychiatry 131: 599–609

Peck D, McGuire R 1988 Behavioural and cognitive therapies. In: Kendell R E, Zealley A K (eds) Companion to Psychiatric Studies, 4th edn. Churchill Livingstone, Edinburgh

132   The concept of schizo-affective disorder was originally introduced by Kasanin who defined it as being an acute psychotic disorder with a mixture of schizophrenic and affective symptoms and having a good prognosis. Until recent times it was very much considered a form of schizophrenia and was classified as such in the 'International Classification of Diseases'. Some, such as Taylor and Abrams, now consider it to be a subtype of affective disorder, while others see it as being different to both schizophrenia and affective disorders and being distinguishable from cycloid psychosis. Brockington and Leff have identified eight different definitions of schizo-affective disorder and they found that the concordance between each is very low. Some definitions emphasise a cross-sectional view while others emphasise the importance of longitudinal pattern of symptoms in making the diagnosis and see it as a mixture of schizophrenic symptoms with an acute onset and having a characteristic course and relatively complete remissions. The validity of any of these concepts has yet to be confirmed. Schizo-affective illness in the first degree relatives of probands with this disorder is rare, but affective disorders are as frequent as in the offspring of probands with an affective disorder. The course, age of onset and response to lithium of schizo-affective illness are variable but more resemble that of bipolar affective disorder than schizophrenia.

Brockington I F, Leff J P 1979 Schizo-affective psychosis: Definitions and incidence. Psychological Medicine 9: 91–99

Taylor M, Abrams R 1973 The phenomenology of mania: A new look at some old patients. Archives of General Psychiatry 29: 520–522

133   Also referred to as the post-traumatic syndrome,
      it consists of symptoms of headache and dizziness
      following what is usually a relatively mild head
      injury. Other features include fatigue, intolerance
      of noise, irritability, emotional instability, insomnia,
      difficulty with memory and concentration and
      minor degrees of intellectual and personality
      disturbances. While it was once considered to be
      a psychogenic disorder and related to compen-
      sation neurosis, recent surveys have found a similar
      constellation of symptoms in both adults and chil-
      dren, irrespective of the question of litigation.
      Various research investigations suggest that the
      syndrome is produced by rotational forces, that
      diffuse damage may be produced in the temporal,
      frontal, mid-brain and limbic areas and that the
      cerebrospinal fluid circulation time is less than
      normal. It would seem that the post-concussional
      syndrome has an organic basis, but that the dur-
      ation of the symptoms may be prolonged in those
      with vulnerable personalities.

Cutting J, McClelland R 1986 Psychiatric
    manifestations of organic illness. In: Hill P, Murray
    R, Thorley A (eds) Essentials of Postgraduate
    Psychiatry 2nd edn. Grune and Stratton, London
Weller M P I 1985 Head Injuries. In:
    Granville–Grossman K (ed) Recent Advances in
    Clinical Psychiatry 5. Churchill Livingstone,
    Edinburgh

134   Prognosis is very varied and depends on complex
      interactions between the individual, the drugs
      abused and socio-economic influences. Mortality
      rates for opiate drug takers are about fifteen times
      that of the non-drug taking population. Estimates
      of mortality from the USA and Britain range from
      16 to 30 per 1,000 per year. Thorley reported that
      approximately one-third of addicts had ceased
      opiate use after seven years. However, Robin's
      survey of Vietnam veterans showed that only 7%
      of a group of heroin users were still dependent
      8–12 months after return to the USA. Pre-service
      drug use was the strongest predictor of continuing
      use. For successful rehabilitation employment is
      seen as crucial while belonging to a minority
      group, having a poor academic performance or a
      criminal record are seen as impediments to
      recovery. In Gordon's study of British Clinics the
      addict's poor academic achievement and criminal
      involvement were the chief obstacles to social
      recovery. Marked criminality rather than continued

addiction was the main deviant behaviour noted in this 10 year follow-up study. ·

Gordon A M 1983 Drug and delinquency. A 10 year follow-up of drug clinic patients. British Journal of Psychiatry 142: 169–173

Robins L N, Halzer J E, Davis D H 1975 Narcotic use in South-East Asia and afterwards. Archives of General Psychiatry 32: 955–961

Stinson G, Oppenheimer E 1982 Heroin addiction: Treatment and control in Britain. Tavistock, London

135 Suicide rates increase with age and are greater in males than females. The rate for single people is twice that of divorced and separated people and 4–5 times higher than that of married persons. Suicide rates show a social class effect with increased rates at both extremes of the economic scale, the greatest increase occurring in social class V, with increases above average in classes I and IV. The increase in social class I is not found in persons under 35 years of age, whereas in the lower social classes the increased rate is particularly marked in this age group. The suicide rate is higher in urban than rural areas, in whites than blacks and in immigrant populations. Other correlates associated include retirement, separation, unemployment, redundancy, poor social support, social isolation, increased social mobility and socially disorganised areas.

Morgan H G 1982 Deliberate self-harm. In: Granville–Grossman K (ed) Recent Advances in Clinical Psychiatry 4. Churchill Livingstone, Edinburgh

Sainsbury P, Jenkins J, Levy A 1980 The social correlates of suicide in Europe. In: Farmer R, Hirsch S (eds) The Suicide Syndrome. Croom Helm, London

136 The aetiology is probably multi-factorial. A neuroleptic induced aetiology has been proposed but it has not been firmly established. Double blind trials have shown that placebo groups have the same frequency of depressive symptoms as active drug recipients and that there is a significant reduction of depressive symptoms when patients are treated with neuroleptics. Depressive symptoms may be an integral part of schizophrenia, as evidenced by the high frequency of depressive symptoms in schizophrenia, irrespective of whether the patient is on neuroleptic

medication or not, their tendency to recur and the fact that they remit rather than increase after treatment has begun. These depressive symptoms tend to be revealed during the remission phase. Post psychotic depression refers to the possibility that depression may occur as the schizophrenic gains insight into his illness and the future prospect of having a chronic relapsing psychoses. Life events such as redundancy, rejection by family and friends and lack of social support may leave the patient particularly vulnerable to depression. Premorbid personality traits may also be important in the aetiology of depression. Depression associated with schizophrenia must be distinguished from 'akinetic depression', a neuroleptic induced extrapyramidal syndrome which resembles depression and responds to anticholinergic drugs.

Knight A, Hirsch S 1981 'Revealed' depression and drug treatment for schizophrenia. Archives of General Psychiatry 38: 806–811

Roy A, Thompson R, Kennedy S 1983 Depression in schizophrenia. British Journal of Psychiatry 142: 465–470

137 A previous act of deliberate self harm is one of the highest predictive factors emphasising the tendency for deliberate self harm behaviour to be self perpetuating. A history of previous psychiatric treatment and having a criminal record are also significant factors. Other correlates associated with repetitious self harm behaviour include drug and alcohol abuse, unemployment, membership of lower social classes, separation from spouse, loss of mother before age 15, regret at surviving the first episode, initial episodes not precipitated by any stress and a diagnosis of sociopathy. Some research workers suggest that being widowed, divorced or separated should also be a positive predictor of repetition. Approximately 20–30% of patients make further attempts at self-harm within twelve months.

Buglass D, Horton J 1974 A scale for predicting subsequent suicidal behaviour. British Journal of Psychiatry 124: 573–578

Kreitman N 1988 Suicide and parasuicide. In: Kendell R E, Zealley A K (eds) Companion to Psychiatric Studies, 4th edn. Churchill Livingstone, Edinburgh

138 In the 1970s self poisoning, particularly with tranquillisers, antidepressants and salicylates accounted for 40% of male and 62% of females suicides.

Trends in recent years have shown a decrease in the number of suicides by poisoning with solid or liquid substances. This may be due to a decrease in barbiturate prescribing. There has been a particularly high rise in male suicide by car exhaust fumes and hanging, strangulation and suffocation. These are now the most common methods of male suicide. Suicide using firearms and explosives also has increased substantially in males over the recent years. Suicides by drowning and jumping from a high place have increased in females. The remarkable overall fall of 34% in the suicide rate in England and Wales during the 1960s has been attributed by many to a fall in the carbon monoxide content in domestic gas. In 1963 this method of suicide accounted for one-third of all deaths while by 1972 this method had virtually disappeared.

Morgan H G 1982 Deliberate self-harm. In: Granville–Grossman K (ed) Recent Advances in Clinical Psychiatry 4. Churchill Livingstone, Edinburgh

McClure G 1984 Trends in suicide rates for England and Wales, 1974–1980. British Journal of Psychiatry 164: 119–126

139 The typical personality changes usually reflect those of frontal lobe damage, but occasionally may be associated with temporal lobe or subcortical lesions. Features include deterioration of manners, lack of awareness of social niceties and the needs of others, suspiciousness, depression and the aggravation of a life long personality foible. Affective blunting and shallowness are common features and may present as gross apathy. Excessive emotional responsiveness may be seen in response to trivial annoyance or as emotional lability. Temporal lobe damage can produce similar personality changes along with depersonalisation and altered sexual activity. In the initial phase of dementia memory disturbance is the usual mode of presentation, but occasionally personality or mood changes are the first to be observed. When only personality is affected the changes are best referred to as 'organic personality change' to distinguish it from dementia.

Cutting J, McClelland R 1986 Psychiatric manifestations of organic illness. In: Hill P, Murray R, Thorley A (eds) Essentials of Postgraduate Psychiatry 2nd edn. Grune and Stratton, London

Lishman W A 1978 Cardinal psychological features of cerebral disorder. In: Organic Psychiatry. Blackwell, Oxford

140 Socio-cultural influences are regarded as major factors in the development of illicit drug dependency. The main social influences relate to a deprived urban environment, anomie with retreatist behaviour in response to failure in achieving ambitions, parental loss or disharmony, ineffective parent-child relationship and parental abuse of drugs and alcohol. Social involvement in a neighbourhood with easy drug availability, low cost and a street culture which surrounds drugs are important factors. Other influences include restricted opportunities for acceptable socialisation, peer group influences toward deviant subcultural activities and association with delinquent groups which provide an anti-social model and can supply drug needs. There is a marked association between opiate dependence and delinquency in notified addicts; some 50% have criminal records that predate their drug abuse. Rapid economic growth is seen as a major precursor of a growing drug problem. Social patterns of drug use have changed in recent years with a shift in use from deprived urban black ghettos to adolescents and young adults of all social classes. Drug abuse now shows a decreasing disparity between the sexes.

Bry B H 1983 Predicting drug abuse: review and reformulation. International Journal of Addictions 18: 223–233
Salmon R, Salmon S 1977 The causes of heroin addiction: a review of the literature. International Journal of the Addictions 12: 679–696

141 Optimal treatment of this syndrome should include adequate fluid replacement, correction of electrolyte imbalance, adequate sedation, replenishing thiamine stores and a careful examination for injury or infection. Agitation is helped by use of a well lit room, adequate explanation of procedures to the patient and minimising environmental disturbance. A wide range of sedative drugs are available including the phenothiazines, butyrophenones, chlormethiazole, benzodiazepines, paraldehyde and propranolol. Drugs of the phenothiazine or butyrophenone group are potentially epileptogenic and their use is preferably accompanied by an anticonvulsant drug such as

phenytoin. Chlordiazepoxide has both sedative and anticonvulsant properties and is generally considered the drug of first choice. Chlormethiazole is widely used but is more addictive than the longer acting benzodiazepines. While the above drugs can be helpful with minor withdrawal symptoms, there is no evidence that they shorten the duration or reduce the mortality of delirium tremens. Correction of the common accompanying metabolic abnormalities such as hypokalaemia, hypoglycaemia, hypomagnesaemia, hypophosphataemia and acidosis may be important. Multivitamin preparations should be administered. A balanced diet is important but a carbohydrate loaded diet may draw on stores of already depleted thiamine stores.

Victor M 1983 Mental disorders due to alcoholism. In: Lader M (ed) Handbook of Psychiatry 2 Mental disorders and somatic illness. Cambridge University Press, Cambridge

142 It is regarded as a form of denial of a very brittle and poor self image or an attempt to 'laugh off' a loss or undesirable events. Manic episodes are seen as a merging of the ego functions of an individual with the superego, so that the energy of the latter provides a righteous self-inflated ego with euphoria and extreme narcissistic behaviour. As the denial of the real view of the self or the loss breaks down, depression results. The theory of 'manic defense' or 'flight into mania' is largely associated with Melanie Klein.

Klein M 1934 A contribution to the psychogenesis of manic-depressive states. In: Jones E (ed) Contributions to Psychoanalysis. Hogarth Press, London
Shur E 1986 Affective disorder: Mania. In: Hill P, Murray R, Thorley A (eds) Essentials of Postgraduate Psychiatry 2nd edn. Grune and Stratton, London

143 They refer to an accelerated rate of thinking and are manifest by 'pressure of speech' and a subjective experience of 'racing thoughts'. The connections between successive thoughts are haphazard and the patient wanders off the point following arbitary connections. Verbal associations such as cliches, proverbs and puns are common and are directed by internal superficial associations. Although connections are often accidental they are usually in themselves fairly obvious, unlike

110

the formal thought disorder seen in schizophrenia. Flight of ideas are typical of mania where they may be so severe that incoherence develops. They are seen in a more ordered fashion in hypomania. They may also occur in schizophrenia, in intoxicated people and in some organic syndromes, particularly those associated with lesions of the hypothalamus. It has been claimed that flight of ideas without pressure of speech can occur in mixed affective states.

Hamilton M (ed) 1984 Fish's clinical psychopathology, 3rd edn. Wright, Bristol

144 Depot treatments simplify the administration of neuroleptics by providing a measure of control over the medication prescribed and a certain knowledge of the medication actually being received by the patient. The extent of patient non-compliance with oral medication ranges from 45% in out-patients to 37% in day patients. With depot medication approximately 5–10% will initially refuse the injection and subsequent non-compliance rates will be 15–20% over a two year period. It is accepted that maintenance therapy reduces psychotic phenomena and socially embarrassing behaviour and significantly aids family relationships. It would seem likely because of the problem of poor compliance that depot medication would prove superior to oral treatment in terms of relapse. However, a number of studies have claimed that depot treatment does not produce superior results. Hypothetically, depot medication may have an advantage in that the injection allows a more constant serum level and allows the drug to initially by-pass the de-activating process of the liver.

Falloon I, Watt D C, Shepherd M 1978 A comparative controlled trial of pimozide and fluphenazine decanoate in the continuation therapy of schizophrenia. Psychological Medicine 8: 59–70
Johnson D A W, Freeman H C 1973 Drug defaulting by patients on long acting phenothiazines. Psychological Medicine 3: 115–119

145 The report should convey a clear account of the extent of the injury and impairment, what effect the disability has had on the person's personality and lifestyle and in what way the quality of life in the future is going to differ from what it would otherwise have been. The first section of the

report should detail the time and place of the examination and specify the length of contact with the patient. All aspects of the injury and its complications, such as skull fractures, haematomas and cerebral infections, the duration of unconsciousness, disorientation, retrograde and post-traumatic amnesia, should be described. Results of skull X-rays, CAT scans and EEG reports and psychometric evaluation of memory and cognitive function should be included. A full description of psychological symptoms and personality changes following the accident will be a central aspect of the report. After the descriptive account the facts must then be interpreted and varying degrees of importance should be attached to the various pieces of evidence. Finally the impact of the degree of disability on the person's current and future quality of life must be presented and this should be examined in the light of the person's age, social circumstances and likely expectations.

Gibbens T C N 1974 Preparing psychiatric court reports. British Journal of Hospital Medicine 12: 278–284
Scott P D 1953 Psychiatric reports for magistrates courts. British Journal of Delinquency 4: 82–98

146   The true incidence of sexual problems is difficult to establish because of differing diagnostic criteria and a bias in reporting and sampling methods. Kinsey reported that 1.6% of his sample had permanent erectile impotence, the incidence increasing with advancing age so that by age 70, 27% had erectile impotence. Some 7% of his sample reported 'more than incidental' erectile dysfunction. The reported prevalence rates of erectile dysfunction in other studies are comparable. He also emphasised the rarity of ejaculatory failure, but his figure of 0.15% is disputed by other workers. Likewise the frequency of premature ejaculation varies from 6% in Kinsey's survey to 36% in other surveys. The incidence of female orgasmic dysfunction has also shown wide variations. A review of various surveys indicates that approximately 20% rarely achieve orgasm, 50% sometimes do and 30% almost always reach orgasm. Kinsey reported that 10% of women in their mid-thirties were incapable of orgasm. Survey of some hospital statistics indicate that the prevalence rate for sexual dysfunction is 20% among out-patients attenders. However, other

surveys report that only 12% of first attenders to a psychiatric clinic require sexual or marital therapy.

Cole M 1985 Sex therapy. A critical appraisal. British Journal of Psychiatry 147: 337–351

Cole M 1985 Sex therapy. A critical appraisal. British Journal of Psychiatry 147: 337–351

Kinsey A, Pomeroy W, Martin C 1948 Sexual behaviour in the human male. Saunders, Philadelphia

Kinsey A, Pomeroy W, Martin C, Gebhard P 1953 Sexual behaviour in the human female. Saunders, Philadelphia

147 The onset in multi-infarct dementia is more acute and it follows a stepwise course with marked fluctuations in contrast to the steady decline of senile dementia. Periods of nocturnal confusion are characteristic and there is relative preservation of personality, retention of insight and depressive symptomatology in multi-infarct dementia. In senile dementia the personality changes occur early and insight is lost. Hypertension, transient ischaemic attacks, focal neurological signs, epileptic seizures and a history of somatic complaints are all more common in vascular dementia. Pathologically the disorders are quite distinct but as both are common in the elderly they can occur simultaneously. The Hachinski Ischaemic Score which is based on a brief inventory of clinical signs and symptoms can be used to assist the distinctions between multi-infarct and senile dementia.

Hachinski V C, Iliff L D, Zilkha E 1975 Cerebral blood flow in dementia. Archives of Neurology 32: 632–637

Lishman W A 1978 Senile dementia, presenile dementia and pseudo-dementia. In: Organic Psychiatry. Blackwell Scientific Publications, Oxford

148 Goldstein, Falloon and Leff have examined the possibility that family intervention may reduce relapse rates following schizophrenic episodes. The nature of the interventions vary but all include some type of social support for the family and various methods to reduce expressed emotion. The educational component contains information for the families about the course, clinical features, particularly the negative symptoms and prognosis, the medication used and its side-effects. It places emphasis on the importance of reducing environ-

mental stress. Problem solving techniques are evaluated with families. Useful strategies are explored and tested with the therapist, or alternatively are tried by family members and re-evaluated later with the therapist. Relatives' groups provide a forum for support and enables relatives to observe and change some of their coping strategies. Aspects of maladaptive communication can be identified in families and intervention strategies made for each family's specific defects in communication skills. Lowering of expressed emotion is one of the prime aims of therapy. Attempts are made to reduce critical comments, over-involvement and hostility. The reduction of face-to-face contact is usually part of the overall package of management. Short of independent living, partial separation can be achieved by arranging day care in day centres or workshops. Patients and relatives are encouraged to join structured social groups outside of the home and to spend their leisure time in different activities. Families' expectations for the patient are identified and carefully modified if unrealistic.

Falloon I, Boyd J, McGill C W, Razani J, Moss H, Gilderman A 1982 Family management in the prevention of exacerbations of schizophrenia. New England Journal of Medicine 306: 1437–1440

Leff J 1985 Family treatment of schizophrenia. In: Granville–Grossman K (ed) Recent Advances in Clinical Psychiatry 5. Churchill Livingstone, Edinburgh

149 In younger children, friendships may be described as partnerships focused on a common activity. Adolescents become more self-conscious and tend to request opinions and use acknowledgements. Same sex friendships are typical of adolescence and these may be accompanied by active homosexual experimentation. Especially in girls, there is an intense quality to friendships in the early and mid-teen years with demands of loyalty and pressure to spend much time together. Boys tend to have friendships scattered through a wider group with less conflicting but more stable relationships. The nature of the adolescent's relationship with their peer group is of paramount importance in assisting or retarding separation from the family. Many adolescents attach themselves firmly to the peer group with whom they identify. These 'gangs' range from the idealistic to the delinquent. Occasionally the adolescent will

noose a gang with aspirations which he knows his parents will consider unsuitable. Same sex peer groups slowly tend to give way to mixed groups by mid adolescence and later a pattern of loosely associated groups of couples begin to develop. In keeping with their greater physical maturity, girls join mixed sex groups at an earlier age.

Rutter M 1979 (ed) Changing youth in a changing society. The Nuffield Provincial Hospital Trust, London

150 While most aggressive behaviour can be under-stood in the context of personality attributes, social adjustment and life's circumstances, in some instances it is directly related to cerebral pathology. Focal lesions such as brain tumours, head injuries, birth traumas, temporal lobe epilepsy and intracranial infections will account for abnormal behaviour in a minority of cases. In those cases where no focal pathology can be iden-tified and an organic factor is suspected, it is thought that there may be a dysfunction within the limbic system. Studies of laboratory animals indicate that stimulation of the amygdaloid nuclei can facilitate aggressive outbursts. The term 'episodic dyscontrol syndrome' has been used to describe those who have aggressive behaviour due to disturbed cerebral physiology and this syn-drome is thought to account for a large proportion of cases with recurring unprovoked aggressive behaviour. The majority of subjects are male, come from disturbed and violent family back-grounds and most have EEG abnormalities similar to those of epilepsy originating from the temporal lobes.

Williams D 1969 Neural factors related to habitual aggression. Brain 92: 503–520

151 The majority have been described by Rooth as immature, timid, obsessional, often with a history of poor sexual performance and a reluctance to accept responsibility. They commonly have over-protective mothers and passive fathers and are inclined to marry women who take over the maternal role. These men usually expose a flaccid penis, feel guilty afterwards and have a good prog-nosis. A minority group, some 20%, have psycho-pathic personalities and exposure is clearly sexual in that they have penile erection and usually masturbate. They show little guilt, many derive

115

sadistic pleasure from the act and they have prognosis. Rooth reported a fairly high associa. with paedophilia and voyeurism but sexual violence was exceptional. Exhibitionists usually expose to pubertal girls, though a minority expose persistently to pre-pubertal girls. Most are careful to avoid identification but some will ensure that they are apprehended. Langevin casts doubts over these generalisations. He states that the personality of the exhibitionist is not abnormal, that they do not have sadistic attitudes towards women, nor do they have undue difficulties in heterosexual relationships and that there is no close association with other sexually deviant behaviour apart from a weak association with voyeurism. Exhibitionism may uncommonly be a presenting feature of organic disease. The majority of people are only charged once, the Court appearance having a strong deterrent effect. The chance of re-conviction increases markedly with a second conviction, particularly for men with previous convictions for non-sexual offences.

Langevin R, Paitich D, Ramsey G, Anderson G, Kamrad J, Pope S, Geller G, Pearl L, Newman S 1979 Experimental studies of the aetiology of genital exhibitionism. Archives of Sexual Behaviour 8: 307–331

Rooth F G 1971 Indecent exposure and exhibitionism. British Journal of Hospital Medicine, April 521–533

Rosen I 1978 Exhibitionism, scoptophilia and voyeurism. In: Rosen I L (ed) Sexual Deviation 2nd edn. Oxford University Press, Oxford

152 They are a set of operational diagnostic criteria which were developed from the Feighner Criteria and provide a means of obtaining replicable samples of patients for research. They contain specific and well identified exclusion and inclusion criteria for each diagnosis. Subsequent to the development of this diagnostic instrument Spitzer and Endicott produced a semi-standardised interview schedule called the Schedule for Affective Disorders and Schizophrenia to be used alongside it. Together they produce a high degree of diagnostic reliability especially for affective disorders and schizophrenia. Anorexia nervosa and organic syndromes are not included in the schedule.

Endicott J, Spitzer R L 1978 A diagnostic interview: The schedule for Affective Disorders and Schizophrenia. Archives of General Psychiatry 35: 837–844

ch
Spitzer R L, Endicott J, Robins E 1978 Research
    Diagnostic Criteria. Archives of General Psychiatry
    35: 773–782

153 Depression, which is severe or resistant to chemo-
    therapy and which has certain features that
    predict a favourable response, is the main indi-
    cation. Endogenous features such as guilt feelings,
    depressive delusions, psychomotor retardation,
    weight loss and early morning wakening are associ-
    ated with a favourable therapeutic response. The
    indications for ECT in the treatment of schizo-
    phrenia are poorly established and since it has
    been superseded by phenothiazines its use is now
    usually confined to cases that also have affective
    symptoms. ECT is generally considered to have
    only a short lived tranquillising effect in mania
    and neuroleptics and lithium are now the treat-
    ments of first choice for this disorder.

Fraser M 1982 ECT and depression. In: ECT, a
    clinical guide. Wiley, Chichester
Fraser C P L 1979 Electroconvulsive therapy: its
    current clinical use. British Journal of Hospital
    Medicine 121: 281–292

154 This term is generally applied to paranoid con-
    ditions that are not associated with a primary
    organic, affective or schizophrenic disorder. In the
    ICD 9 system of classification, 'category 297.0
    paranoid state simple' consists of a psychosis in
    which paranoid delusions are the main symptom;
    category 297 also includes paranoia, paraphrenia
    and induced psychoses. DSM III criteria for
    paranoid disorders include paranoid delusions
    persisting for at least one week without prominent
    hallucinations. ICD 9 differs from DSM III in
    that it includes acute paranoid reaction and
    psychogenic paranoid psychoses. Differentiation
    of paranoid states from paranoid schizophrenia
    and severe paranoid personality can be difficult as
    the boundaries of these disorders are unclear.

American Psychiatric Association 1980 Diagnostic and
    Statistical Manual of Mental Disorder 3rd edn.
    Washington DC
World Health Organisation 1978 International
    Classification of Diseases 9th edn. World Health
    Organisation, Geneva

155 The main feature is a grossly disturbed eating
    pattern, alternating between excessive eating and

strict dietary control. The quantity of food eaten during a binge is usually enormous and it generally consists of carbohydrates and 'fattening' foods. Many patients report loss of control over their eating, the binges are usually secretive and may vary from a few times weekly to several times a day. Initially a patient feels relief from tension during the binge but inevitably feelings of guilt, depression and self-disgust are experienced. Binging is followed by self-induced vomiting, often with purgative and diuretic abuse. Many of these patients have a morbid fear of fatness but generally their body weight fluctuates within the normal range. The patient is almost constantly preoccupied with distressing thoughts of food. Depressive symptoms, worthlessness and suicidal ideation are common. The bulimic person is generally described as outgoing, socially competent, sexually experienced and industrious. A minority describe drug and alcohol abuse and promiscuity. Many patients develop a bulimic disorder within a year of onset of anorexic symptoms. In others the interval may be longer or there may be no previous history of anorexia nervosa. Females are more commonly affected than males. Physical complications include menstrual irregularities, cardiac arrythmias, gastric abnormalities, tetany, dental erosion, steatorrhoea, salivary gland enlargement, renal change and epileptic seizures.

Fairburn C 1983 Bulimia nervosa. British Journal of Hospital Medicine 32: 537–542
Palmer R 1982 Anorexia nervosa. In: Granville–Grossman, K (eds) Recent Advances in Clinical Psychiatry 4. Churchill Livingstone, Edinburgh

156 In-patient hospital suicide accounts for 5% of annual suicidal deaths. However, less than 50% commit suicide actually within the hospital, the rest kill themselves on a pass or weekend leave. One survey found that the suicide risk was highest for both sexes in the first week of admission. In-patients with affective disorders seem to have the greatest risk, being up to 5 times greater than in-patients with schizophrenia. In general, studies report that the diagnosis of depressive psychosis carries the greatest risk with females having a greater risk than males. Environmental factors which may influence the occurrence of suicide include poor communication between staff and patient, low staff morale, absence of consultants,

employment of locums and plans for discharge of long term patients. Times of staff rotation are periods associated with in-patient suicides and 'epidemics' of suicide are associated with periods of change in treatment management policy, staff disorganisation and staff demoralisation.

Crammer J L 1984 The special characteristics of suicide in hospital in-patients. British Journal of Psychiatry 145: 460–476

157 This is a disorder of the stream of thought in which the patient experiences his train of thought being stopped and a new one begin and it bears no relationship to the previous thought. In patients who retain some insight this sudden 'blank' may be a frightening experience. When thought blocking is well marked it is almost diagnostic of schizophrenia. However, it is important to realise that the tired and anxious person may have difficulty maintaining the stream of thought and may appear to block. Thought block must also be distinguished from inhibition of thinking which may occur in depressive states.

Hamilton M (ed) 1984 Fish's clinical psychopathology, 3rd edn. Wright, Bristol

158 The assessment should aim to confirm or refute the diagnosis and establish a possible cause when dementia is present. A complete and well documented history is essential for the differential diagnosis of dementia. The history of symptom development may contain clues of great significance and aspects such as the mode of onset, whether acute or insidious, the speed of deterioration, the age of onset and the form of the presenting symptoms should be enquired about. Alzheimer's disease tends to present with personality deterioration as a marked feature and shows a global progressive deterioration while multi-infarct dementia may present with a step wise deterioration with focal neurological signs. Certain symptoms are of particular importance such as epileptic seizures, visual disturbances, speech and language defects and weight loss. A past psychiatric, medical and surgical history is taken. A detailed account of all medications being taken is noted, both prescribed and over the counter drugs. Enquiries should be made of a family history of organic and functional illness and a careful search for alcohol abuse both in the

patient's and the family's history. It is essential to assess the patient's mental state with particular emphasis on cognitive performance and mood. There are many questionnaires in general use which assess orientation, past memory for general and personal events and recent memory. A physical examination may give clues to the diagnosis; hypertension and evidence of arteriosclerotic changes may suggest a multi-infarct dementia, cranial nerves may be damaged if a tumour is the cause, rigidity and tremor may be evidence of the presence of Parkinson's disease and a disturbed gait and urinary incontinence may indicate a diagnosis of normal pressure hydrocephalus.

Lishman W A 1978 (ed) Senile dementia, presenile dementia and pseudodementia. In: Organic Psychiatry. Blackwell, Oxford

159   Some 97% of Down's syndrome cases are of the trisomy-G type and are due to non-disjunction, which is associated with increasing maternal age. Mosaicism is found in 2–3% of cases and translocation is a relatively uncommon form of chromosomal abnormality in Down's syndrome. The translocations arise when chromosome No. 21 is translocated onto another chromosome, the most common being a G/D translocation with chromosome No. 14 and a G/G translocation with chromosome No. 22.

Nelson Textbook of Paediatrics 1983 12th edn. Vaughan V, McKay R, Behrmann R (eds) Saunders, London

160   The principal party to physical abuse is generally the primary caretaker and so the majority are the mothers of the affected children. They tend to be socially isolated and surveys indicate that about half of the fathers are unemployed. Though much of the data is retrospective or relies on individual case reports, it seems likely that in many instances the abusing parent will also have been abused as a child. Characteristically the parent has limited empathy for the child, exhibits a 'role reversal' whereby the child is expected unreasonably to care for the parent's dependency needs and there may be other features of criminal behaviour. Indeed, it is strongly suggested that among a malignant hardcore of abusing parents, child

abuse is only one aspect of more generally violent behaviour.

Mrazek D, Mrazek M 1985 Child maltreatment. In: Rutter M, Hersov L (eds) Child and Adolescent Psychiatry. Modern Approaches 2nd edn. Blackwell, Oxford

Smith S, Kunjukrishnan R 1985 Child abuse, perspectives on treatment and research. In: The Psychiatric Clinics of North America. Child Psychiatry December 1985 Saunders, Philadelphia

161 Excessive use of cannabis over long periods of time has been reported to lead to psychotic states, the 'amotivational syndrome' and intellectual and social deterioration. An acute psychotic state which resolves within days of stopping the drug is characterised by paranoid delusions and hallucinations. The relationship of cannabis use to chronic psychotic states remains unproved but the evidence suggests some connection. 'Flashbacks' may occur after stopping the drug. The 'amotivational syndrome' is characterised by apathy, self-neglect, loss of ambition and inactivity. The association between this syndrome and prolonged use of cannabis has been based on a large number of clinical observations, but the features have not been satisfactorily reproduced under experimental conditions. Earlier reports of cerebral atrophy in chronic users, as detected by air encephalography, have not been confirmed by recent studies using computerised axial tomography. Cannabis has also been implicated in producing lung damage, cardiac complications, low sperm count, decreased serum levels of testosterone, impaired sexual performance, ovulatory dysfunction, infertility and foetal abnormalities.

Granville–Grossman K 1979 Psychiatric aspects of cannabis abuse. In: Granville–Grossman K (ed) Recent Advances in Clinical Psychiatry. Churchill Livingstone, Edinburgh

Lishman W A 1978 Toxic disorders. In: Organic Psychiatry Blackwell, Oxford

162 Bipolar mood patterns have been categorised into bipolar I and II, and more recently into bipolar III. The bipolar I group refers to those with very definite and severe manic and depressive episodes, while bipolar II patients are those who have had treatment for depression, but only have short and relatively mild hypomanic episodes. The bipolar III category, also known as unipolar II, have

definite episodes of depression, a family history of bipolar disorder and have had hypomanic moods in response to antidepressant chemotherapy. Bipolar I and II subtypes have been further divided on the basis of the temporal sequence of depression and mania, that is, into the 'mania—depression—interval' course and the 'depression—mania—interval' course. Some bipolar mood changes follow a 'continuous cycle' and to this belong 'rapid cyclers', those with prolonged depressions and short manic spells and a heterogenous group. Patients in the 'continuous cycle' group are only free from depression or elation for a few weeks at most in any one year.

Kukopulos A, Reginaldi D 1980 Recurrences of manic-depressive episodes during lithium treatment. In: Johnson F N (ed) Handbook of Lithium Therapy. M T P Press, Lancaster

Perris C 1982 The distinction between bipolar and unipolar depressive disorders. In: Paykel E S (ed) Handbook of Affective Disorders. Churchill Livingstone, Edinburgh

163 Surveys of autopsy material from psychiatric hospitals have shown that the chance of finding a cerebral tumour is greater than in post-mortem studies in general hospitals, 3.7% compared to 2.4%, and some two-thirds are only diagnosed at autopsy. The type and severity of the mental symptoms are dependent on the site, rate of growth and invasiveness of the tumour. The more rapidly expanding lesions produce acute impairment of consciousness while the more slowly growing meningiomas, which constitute some 30% of tumours in surveys of psychiatric hospitals compared to half that number in general hospitals, present with subtle personality changes or cognitive impairment. Conditions which are most likely to be diagnosed are presenile and senile dementia, cerebral atherosclerosis, epilepsy and to a lesser extent schizophrenia, affective disorders and neurotic states.

Lishman W A 1978 Cerebral tumours. In: Organic Psychiatry. Blackwell, Oxford

164 The first aspect of management is to establish whether it is a primary or secondary phenomenon. Depersonalisation may be a symptom of an anxiety, phobic or depressive illness or a prodromal feature of schizophrenia and the treat-

ment in these instances is directed at the primary disorder. Intoxication with psychomimetic drugs, temporal lobe epilepsy, hypoglycaemia, hypercalcaemia and other metabolic and organic disorders can produce symptoms of depersonalisation and as such an EEG recording and metabolic screening are recommended. Treatment of the primary disorder involves explaining to the patient that you understand the symptoms, as they almost invariably feel misunderstood, and giving ongoing supportive psychotherapy. Avoidance of precipiting factors such as fatigue, anxiety and illicit drugs may be helpful. Specific treatment is not available. In instances where the onset was related to a particular life event, a psychotherapeutic approach can be useful. Antidepressant medication, particularly the monoamine-oxidase inhibitors often ameliorate the symptoms. Phenothiazines and electroconvulsive therapy can intensify symptoms and should be avoided.

Sedman G 1970 Theories of depersonalisation: A reappraisal. British Journal of Psychiatry 117: 1–14
Snaith P 1980 Anxiety and phobic neurosis. In: Clinical Neurosis. Oxford University Press, Oxford

165 Reports of the frequency of depression vary widely according to the methods used, but most studies have shown it to be common in schizophrenia. Hirsch found that 15% of chronic schizophrenics in out-patients required antidepressant medication and that about one-half had depression for some time during the six months following discharge. Prospective studies indicate that for chronic schizophrenic patients on regular neuroleptic medication the risk of an episode of depression was over three times the risk of an acute schizophrenic relapse, and over a two year period the total duration of morbidity from depression was more than twice the duration of morbidity from acute schizophrenic symptoms. Depressive symptoms may develop prior to an acute schizophrenic relapse, during the relapse and following the psychotic disorder. It may also occur following long periods in remission.

Johnson D 1986 Depressive symptoms in schizophrenia: Some observations on the frequency, morbidity and possible causes. In: Kerr A, Snaith P (eds) Contemporary Issues in Schizophrenia Gaskell Psychiatry Series
Roy A 1986 (ed) Depression, attempted suicide and suicide in patients with chronic schizophrenia. In:

The Psychiatric Clinics of North America.
Schizophrenia. March 1986 195–205. Saunders,
Philadelphia

166 Assessment of the symptom of enuresis should
always include assessment of the child's physical,
cognitive and emotional development and the
family's circumstances. A carefully collected mid-
stream specimen of urine should be examined for
white cells and proteins and cultured. Generally
no other urological examination is required.
Treatment is preceded by a period of observation
using star charts. Rewards for dry nights during
this period may have a beneficial effect. The bell
and pad method can result in a permanent cure
in a high proportion of cases and is therefore the
method of choice. This device sounds a buzzer
which wakens the child when he wets the sheet.
Approximately 30% of children are dry within
three months, though about one-third of children
relapse when the treatment is stopped. Relapses
can be reduced by a period of over-learning and
intermittent reinforcement. A major problem with
the bell and pad is the high drop out rate before
treatment is effective. This chiefly results from
irritation with false alarms, inability to understand
or carry out instructions or failure of the buzzer
to wake the child. Tricyclic antidepressant drugs
are generally not indicated because of the success
rate of behavioural methods and the side effects
and high relapse rate associated with drugs.
However, because of their simplicity of use and
rapidity of action, they are useful when it is
important to achieve an immediate short term
effect such as when the child is going on holiday
or to relieve stresses in the family. For those children who wet during the day a full psychiatric,
intellectual and environmental assessment is
required. It is especially important to culture the
urine as some 50% have a urinary infection and
further urological investigation may be indicated.
Various behavioural techniques have been used
such as habit training, over correction and operant
reinforcement of appropriate elimination. The
more intensive programmes have been used in
mentally retarded children with enuresis.

Dische S 1973 Treatment of enuresis with an enuresis
    alarm. In: Kolvin I, MacKeith R C, Meadow S R
    (eds) Bladder Control and Enuresis Clinical
    Development Medicine, 48–49. Simp Heinemann,
    London

Taylor E 1983 Disturbance of toilet function. In:
Russell G, Hersov L Handbook of Psychiatry 4.
The neuroses and personality disorder. Cambridge
University Press, Cambridge

167 A haemoglobin estimation, white cell count, blood
film, an ESR, general blood biochemical screen
and serological tests will help identify the different
causes of dementia. Blood count may reveal
anaemia, macrocytosis, a B12 or folate deficiency,
or indicate alcohol abuse. Connective tissue
disease or cranial arteritis would be suspected with
a raised erythrocyte sedimentation rate. Urea,
electrolyte and liver function tests might reveal
renal or hepatocellular impairment and raised
gamma glutamyl transferase may be an indicator
of alcohol abuse. If neurosphyilis is considered
serological tests such as VDRL and TPI would be
helpful as would cerebrospinal fluid analysis.
Hypothyroidism may be diagnosed by low serum
thyroxine and raised thyroid stimulating hormone
levels. Chest and skull X-rays may help identify
cardiac enlargement or bronchial lesions, calcified
masses, bony erosions or demonstrate pineal shift.
The contribution of cardiac arrythmias, valvular
and ischaemic heart disease to these clinical
features of the dementia may be gleaned from an
ECG. The EEG may show diffuse slowing in
primary cerebral atrophies or metabolic encephalopathies or may show focal changes where there
is a space occupying lesion. Computerised
tomography can demonstrate ventricular dilation,
focal lesions such as tumours, infarcts or haematomas and can be useful adjuncts alongside the
clinical findings. It is recommended that all
instances of dementia under the age of sixty-five
should be scanned. In special circumstances a
carotid or cerebral angiogram may be necessary
to identify vascular stenosis or occlusion.

Granville–Grossman K 1986 (ed.) Recent Advances in
Psychogeriatrics. Churchill Livingstone, Edinburgh
Lewis S 1986 CT scanning in psychiatry. British
Journal Hospital Medicine 35: 143

168 The distinction is often impossible to establish
unless the patient is observed over a period of
time. In pseudodementia the families usually
complain of the memory and cognitive problems
and can date the onset of symptoms and outline
their progression. The relatives of those with true

dementia often find the onset of symptoms difficult to date. The pseudodements forcibly complain of cognitive and performance difficulties in contrast to the frequent anosognosia seen in dementia. Patients with pseudodements generally resent examination and give 'don't know' answers, while those with dementia do their best, often exhibiting the 'catastrophic' reaction. Clearly defined defects of temperoparietal functions such as apraxias, dysphasias and R–L discrimination are more often absent in pseudodementia. Memory loss in pseudodementia is generally equally severe for remote and recent events, but is greater for recent memory in the cerebral organic disorder. A previous history or positive family history for depression, an onset of depressive symptoms before memory difficulties and the presence of early morning wakening with guilt and worthlessness and diurnal variation in symptoms all suggest a depressive aetiology. Pseudodementia often shows marked variability in performance on tasks of similar difficulties, have differences on detailed testing of memory function to that of dementia and the symptoms are generally of shorter duration and show rapid progression.

Arie T 1982 Pseudodementia. British Medical Journal 286: 1301–1302
Psychological Medicine 1985 (Editorial) Depression and dementia: The multi-faceted relationship, 227–236.

169 They are complex behavioural and experiental manifestations of ongoing epileptic discharge. They have an abrupt onset, are frequently preceded by the aural features of a grand mal fit and may replace the fit proper or be followed by a grand mal seizure. Psychomotor seizures need to be distinguished from postictal phenomena where there is disturbed cerebral activity unrelated to ongoing seizure activity. The term 'psychomotor seizure' is often used synonomously with epileptic equivalents, psychomotor attacks, epileptic automatisms, fugues and twilight states. Epileptic automatisms are periods of continuous electrical disturbance in the EEG recording, during or immediately before a seizure, in which the subject maintains posture and is able to perform motor tasks of varying complexity without being aware of what is happening. The majority last a few seconds to several minutes and they occasionally terminate with a grand mal

seizure. The seizure focus is usually in the medial temporal lobe but it can arise in the frontal grey matter. Epileptic fugue states are rare occurrences, characterised by lengthy disturbances lasting hours to days during which the person tends to wander away in a perplexed manner. Twilight epileptic states describe the abnormal subjective experience due to electrical discharge rather than the motor manifestations. They last from an hour to a week, consciousness is impaired and the subject can appear muddled. Anger, panic, anxiety and ecstasy are the most common experiences but visual hallucinations can also occur. They culminate in a fit more often than the epileptic automatisms and the subject can only describe the experience afterwards.

Lishman W A 1978 Epilepsy. In: Organic Psychiatry. Blackwell, Oxford

170 Lesions in this area affect personality and neurological function rather than cognitive ability and often the first sign is a lessening of personality reserve, gradually leading to a complete lack of inhibition. The patient may be indiscreet and tactless, have poor judgement and show a lapse in social and ethical standards. Some have a giddy, prankish manner with an empty, fatuous euphoria, while others are apathetic, lack initiative, have impaired concentration to an extent that may mimic dementia and in the extreme may lapse into a catatonic like state. The former features are associated with lesions of the orbital undersurface and the latter with damage of the convex lateral surface of the frontal lobes. Formal tests of intelligence show little evidence of cognitive impairment but special tests show evidence of poor abstracting ability and difficulty in changing forms of reference. Loss of urinary sphincter control is often an early sign of a frontal lesion and is a useful diagnostic pointer. Other neurological signs are a contralateral spastic paresis, especially of the face, hypertonic reflexes, extensor plantar responses, dysphasia, optic tract damage and anosmia.

Lishman W A 1978 Symptoms and syndromes with regional affiliations. In: Organic Psychiatry Blackwell, Oxford
Bond M R 1988 Organic disorders. In: Kendell R E, Zealley A K (eds) Companion to Psychiatric Studies, 4th edn. Churchill Livingstone, Edinburgh

171 Most studies estimate that approximately 10% of schizophrenics kill themselves and some 20% make suicide attempts. Schizophrenics who kill themselves tend to be under the age of forty-five; as many as 80% are male. A clinical course characterised by many exacerbations, remissions and frequent hospitalisations increases the suicide risk. These patients experience severe functional deterioration yet retain a realistic awareness of the effects of their psychopathology. Changes in clinical course precipitate suicide and the period of clinical improvement following relapse is a particularly vulnerable time. Some 30% of suicides occur within one month of discharge from hospital and 50% within three months. Suicide occurred more frequently during periods of depression and hopelessness than active psychosis. Signs of severe agitation and excessive treatment dependence during hospitalisations are ominous signs. Previous suicidal behaviour increases the risk. Suicide has also been related to social isolation in general and to lack of familial support in particular. Surveys have failed to show any direct causal relationship between neuroleptic medication and suicide in schizophrenia.

Roy A 1982 Suicide in chronic schizophrenia. British Journal of Psychiatry 141: 171–177

Roy A 1986 (ed) Depression, attempted suicide and suicide in patients with chronic schizophrenia. In: The Psychiatric Clinics of North America March 1986 193–205. Saunders, Philadelphia

172 Research studies indicate that social class is not an aetiological factor in development of schizophrenia. Faris and Dunham in 1939 showed the incidence of schizophrenia to be higher in central areas of larger cities as compared to wealthier residential suburbs. Hare in 1956 suggested that this was due to a pre-psychotic drift to areas of social isolation and increased tolerance of peculiar behaviour. Goldberg and Morrison emphasised the importance of the 'downward social drift'. They found an excess of schizophrenics in social class V but showed the social class distribution of the fathers of schizophrenics to be similar to that of the general population. Other authors have confirmed this work. Studies of particular cases have generally shown that schizophrenics either fall in occupational level because of their illness or never achieve their expected potential because of early onset of the illness.

Fish F J 1984 Fish's schizophrenia 3rd edn. Hamilton
    M. (ed) Wright, Bristol
Smith A 1986 General and historical concepts:
    Overview. In: Kerr A, Snaith P (eds) Contemporary
    Issues in Psychiatry. Gaskell Psychiatry Series

173 The main features of this syndrome are multiple
motor and vocal tics with coprolalia, coproxia
and palilalia. Simple motor tics are the usual
initial presenting symptom, but for 30% vocal tics
are the first manifestation and 6% present with
coprolalia. The onset is usually between the ages
of 2 and 15. The aetiology is unknown but
biochemical and physiological factors have been
implicated in addition to learning influences,
environmental contingencies and emotional stresses.
Its course tends to be one of chronic fluctuations
in severity with a shifting pattern of tics. Behavioural management, psychotherapeutic strategies
and drug treatment have all been recommended.
The behavioural techniques employed are relaxation training, massed practice and operant conditioning. However, their efficacy remains uncertain.
Haloperidol seems to produce a more specific
effect than simple relaxation and its benefits may
be associated with its dystonic side effects and
dopamine blocking actions. Recent reviews of its
efficacy suggest that there is substantial improvements in at least two-thirds of cases and that doses
of 0.5 to 1.5 tds are usually sufficient in children.
Pimozide may be equally effective and in low
doses has relatively few side effects. Clonidine
seems to be effective in a small proportion of
patients.

Hill P 1986 Child psychiatry. In: Hill P, Murray R,
    Thorley A (eds) Essentials of Postgraduate
    Psychiatry 2nd edn. Grune and Stratton, London

174 Attention should be paid to evaluation of
suicidal risk, risk of repetition and identification
of psychiatric disorder. A detailed account of the
act—the preceding events and circumstances
surrounding the act should be sought. One should
examine the patient's current social and interpersonal situation, alcohol and drug consumption and
physical state. A review of the patient's previous
coping abilities and his current coping resources
will help in evaluation. A relevant family and
personal history, premorbid personality assessment and relevant past psychiatric history should

be obtained. A detailed mental state examination is essential. This should include assessment of past suicide attempts and current suicidal ideations. As patients in a crisis are often more self deprecatory and pessimistic than usual, a family or marital interview is often the most reliable means of evaluating interpersonal conflicts and patients' coping abilities. A decision regarding follow up after this assessment should be made such as referral to family doctor, psychiatric or social services. This decision should be fully discussed and agreed with the patient.

Hawton K, Catalan J 1981 Psychiatric management of attempted suicide patients. British Journal of Hospital Medicine 25: 365–372

175 This term is usually applied to a new word formation produced by schizophrenics and it needs to be distinguished from the distorted word structure of aphasic patients. These idiosyncratic words may be entirely new words whose derivation cannot be understood, or be a word which has been created by compressing together other existing words. Occasionally a neologism is an accepted word that is used in a special way by the patient. Kleist considers that neologisms are part of thought disorder. In other patients the neologisms are part of a delusional experience or arise from auditory hallucinations. Neologisms in catatonics may be mannerisms or stereotypies.

Hamilton M 1984 (ed) Fish's clinical psychopathology, 3rd edn. Wright, Bristol

176 The DSM II is a descriptive diagnostic manual while the DSM III employs operational definitions. The latter is an extension of the Research Diagnostic Criteria which provides operational definitions for all diagnostic categories. It is primarily intended for use in clinical practice, but it is also a reliable research instrument. It employs a multi-axial classification: psychiatric syndromes are described on axis I, personality and developmental disorders on axis II, physical disorders on axis III, psychosocial stressors on IV and highest level of functioning on axis V. The DSM III is gradually gaining acceptance in clinical practice in the USA and it provides the best hope for an internationally acceptable operational diagnostic instrument.

Helzer J E 1983 Standardized interviews in psychiatry. Psychiatric Developments 2: 161–178

Spitzer R L, Williams J B W, Skodol A E 1980 DSM III: The major achievements and an overview. American Journal of Psychiatry 137: 151–164

177 Personality disorders are encountered in a minority of epileptics but it seems doubtful that there is a specific 'epileptic personality'. Descriptions from the older literature of a specific personality type probably detailed a mixture of institutional neurosis and substantial brain damage. Parental and sibling attitudes, brain lesions, ictal and interictal discharges and anticonvulsant drugs can contribute to the personality disturbance. While those with petit mal tend to have neurotic problems and to be relatively passive, those with temporal lobe seizures are explosive, impulsive, moody, histrionic and antisocial. Anticonvulsant drugs which result in better control of fits usually lead to greater emotional stability. However, with increasing doses of these drugs behaviour disturbances may result from their toxic effects, despite a reduction in the frequency of convulsions.

Lishman W A 1978 Epilepsy. In: Organic Psychiatry. Blackwell, London

Ounsted C, Lindsay J 1981 Long term outcome of temporal lobe epilepsy in childhood. In: Reynolds E H, Trimble M R (eds) Epilepsy and Psychiatry. Churchill Livingstone, Edinburgh

178 The major withdrawal symptom is anxiety with its somatic accompaniments. These include nausea, sweating, sleep disturbance, anorexia, fatigue, tremor, muscular pains and dysphoria. Other symptoms include perceptual disturbances, such as depersonalisation, hypersensitivity to all sensory stimuli, false perception of movement, numbness and psychotic symptoms such as paranoid delusions and visual hallucinations. Ataxia and grand mal convulsions may also occur. The symptoms begin two to three days following cessation of short-acting drugs and between seven to ten days after stopping long acting agents. None of the symptoms are pathognomonic of this syndrome and their nature and severity appear to be independent of dosage. The severity of the symptoms seems greater in patients with a rapid

fall in plasma concentration levels and in those patients with passive-dependent personalities.

Hallstrom C, Lader M H 1981 Benzodiazepine withdrawal phenomena. International Pharmacopsychiatry 16: 235–244
Tyrer P 1984 Identification and management of benzodiazepine dependence. Postgraduate Medical Journal 60 (2): 41–46

179 Studies, with general population controls, show that depressed patients report almost three times as many life events as the matched controls in the six months before the onset of depression. The type of events experienced are of the loss variety: death, marital separation, loss of self-esteem and family friction. Several studies have found that depressive illnesses which were preceded by severe life events showed only slight symptom differences from depressions which were not precipitated by such factors. Even those with markedly endogenous depressive features were frequently found to have had major stressful events. This is thought to indicate that stress can unleash a personality or genetic predisposition to depression and that it is not a necessary prelude to depression in those with a particularly strong familial history of affective disorders.

Brown G W, Harris T O, Copeland J R 1977 Depression and loss. British Journal of Psychiatry 130: 1–18
Paykel E S 1982 Life events and early environment. In: Paykel E S (ed) Handbook of Affective Disorders. Churchill Livingstone, Edinburgh

180 The majority of soilers can be categorised into three groups. In one group are those who fail to develop bowel control and they are younger children who pass normal stools into their clothes, as though into nappies. They tend to come from homes of socially disadvantaged families, with poor supervision and are often poorly trained in a number of ways. A few children may be mentally retarded, or have other problems such as physical clumsiness or delay in language development. In the second group there are again normally formed stools, but bowel control breaks down under stress and stools are deposited often in very inappropriate places. Acute stress such as separation from parents, change of school or

bereavement may result in a temporary loss of control. Chronic stress such as marital disharmony, family instability and punitive management may be associated with a relatively intractable disorder with the stool often being placed where it will cause the most irritation. In the third group the stools are abnormal in that they are usually excessively fluid or very hard. The former may be due to an inflammatory bowel disorder or severe anxiety. Severe constipation with overflow may result from local pathology such as a painful anal fissure or Hirschsprung's disease, but it may also be a result of psychological factors such as anxiety centred around toilet training or a constant struggle between mother and child. Another variety of soiling relates to inappropriate toileting behaviour in the form of a 'toilet phobia'. Night time soiling may be due to anal masturbation but this is rare.

Hersov L 1985 Faecal soiling. In: Rutter M, Hersov L (eds) Clinical and Adolescent Psychiatry, 2nd edn. Blackwell, Oxford

181 This term is used to describe a group of disorders which present clinically with a picture resembling organic dementia but are functional in aetiology. Pseudodementia can be distinguished from dementia proper by its clinical features, reversibility, lack of progression and functional aetiology. Distinctions are mainly made on clinical grounds and to a lesser extent on psychological, radiological and laboratory investigations. The causes of these pseudodementias are predominantly forms of depressive illness, but other causes include the Ganser syndrome, simulated dementia and hysterical pseudodementia. Rarer causes are hypomania, schizophrenia, severe obsessional and anxiety states and drug toxicity.

Lishman W A 1978 Senile dementia, presenile dementia and pseudodementia. In: Organic Psychiatry. Blackwell, Oxford
Psychological Medicine 1985 Editorial. Depression and dementia: The multi-faceted relationship. 15: 227–236

182 Psychological causes are the most common with organic factors probably being implicated in less than 10% of cases. Kaplan distinguishes four factors as immediate causes of the dysfunction. These are failure to engage in effective sexual behaviour, to

ignorance or anxiety, fear of failure, spectatoring or failure to communicate. At a more fundamental level, the aetiology of erectile dysfunction is related to intrapsychic and interpersonal conflicts. The intrapsychic conflicts may arise from guilt or sexual anxieties based on early restrictive upbringing or disturbed parental relationships. Anger, guilt, lack of trust, power struggles or fear of rejection may be the result of interpersonal conflicts and may lead to sexual dysfunction. Organic causes, while rare, are many. They include: general physical illness, particularly hepatic and renal disease, diabetes and other endocrine disorders such as hypopituitarism and hypothyroidism. Other causes include disseminated sclerosis and other neurological disorders, peripheral arterial disease and local penile disorders. Drugs which may cause impotence include phenothiazines, tricyclic antidepressants, anticholinergics, digoxin, cimetidine, diuretics, some antihypertensives, alcohol and opiates. Surgical causes usually involve impairment of the nerve supply as in vascular surgery or radical prostatectomy.

Bancroft J 1983 Human sexuality and its problems. Churchill Livingstone, Edinburgh
Kaplan H S 1978 The new sex therapy. Ballière Tindall and Peregrine Books, London

183   Day hospitals provide a link between in-patient and domiciliary care and are used by both services. It serves many functions: assessment of physical, psychological and social needs of the elderly person and their family, and provides treatment and support. Day hospital support for the elderly person living at home is generally dependent on the presence of a relative at home. For the elderly person day care offers the advantage of being able to live at home despite many disabilities. For the family it offers an opportunity for ordinary activities to continue without the constant worry and need for supervision of the elderly person. Day hospitals help maintain individuals in the community for as long as possible. They provide social contact, a proper nutritional programme for isolated elderly and occupational therapy at the hospitals offer occupation and retention of basic skills.

Levy R, Post F 1982 (eds) The psychiatry of late life. Blackwell, Oxford

184   Psychotic symptoms have a complex relationship
       with epilepsy. In some the predominant feature
       is confusion and impairment of consciousness with
       minimal or absent schizophreniform features,
       these states representing the cerebral dysrhyth-
       mias associated with ictal automatisms, petit mal
       and post-ictal confusional episodes. Such features
       last for minutes to hours, or very occasionally for
       days. In the next 'syndrome', which is particularly
       related to temporal lobe epilepsy, the patient
       presents with marked confusion, paranoid de-
       lusions, depression and auditory and visual hal-
       lucinations. The impairment of consciousness may
       not be obvious at the time and the episode often
       lasts days to weeks. It is differentiated from schizo-
       phrenia by the presence of impaired conscious-
       ness. Then there are two distinct schizophrenic
       like syndromes occurring in clear consciousness
       associated with epilepsy. One is a transient
       psychotic episode lasting from days to weeks,
       during which there is normalization of the elec-
       troencephalogram recording. The other is a
       chronic paranoid hallucinatory state occurring in
       those with temporal lobe epilepsy and is indistin-
       guishable from paranoid schizophrenia. It tends
       to start on average fourteen years after the onset
       of the epilepsy, often when the fits are in abeyance
       and runs a variable course. In many cases dull-
       ness, perseveration and memory impairment
       supervene at a later stage.

       Perez M, Trimble M 1980 Epileptic psychosis:
           Diagnostic comparison with process schizophrenia.
           British Journal of Psychiatry 137: 245–249
       Slater E, Beard A W, Clithero E 1963 The
           schizophrenia-like psychoses of epilepsy. British
           Journal of Psychiatry 109: 95–105

185   The prevalence rates for depression vary with the
       diagnostic criteria being used and will be influ-
       enced by whether the survey is based on a
       community, a general practise, or a psychiatric
       treatment facility sample. With the development
       of reliable and well defined criteria, such as the
       Research Diagnostic Criteria or the DSM III,
       some consensus on the prevalence of depressive
       disorders is beginning to emerge. The point
       prevalence of depressive symptoms, not suf-
       ficiently severe to reach operational criteria for
       depression, seems to range between 13 and 20%
       of the population while the point prevalence for
       depressive disorders is about 3% for men and

between 5 and 9% for women. The morbid risk of bipolar disorders in industrialised nations is approximately 0.8%.

Boyd J H, Weissman M M 1982 Epidemiology. In: Paykel E S (ed) Handbook of Affective Disorders. Churchill Livingstone, Edinburgh

Weissman M M, Myers J K 1978 Affective disorders in a USA urban community. Archives of General Psychiatry 35: 1304–1311

186 Bruising on the lower back, buttocks, face, ear lobes or upper lip may result from excessive chastisement. Oral injuries such as a torn frenulum might suggest forced feeding. Straps or sticks may leave tell-tale parallel marks. Sexual abuse may be indicated by genital bruises, but penile injuries can be due to sadistic attempts to deal with enuresis. Ocular injuries such as acute hyphaema, traumatic cataract and retinal detachment are not unusual. Retinal haemorrhage may be associated with subdural haemorrhage and these may actually occur without signs of external injury. Clinical evidence of increased intracranial pressure or focal neurological signs should be sought. Some 4 to 8% of hospitalised children with burns and 25% of those with tap water scalds have been abused. Cigarette burns and burning or branding with hot metal objects are other forms of abuse. Scalds with a 'high water mark' are especially suspicious of 'dunking'. Abdominal injuries resulting from abuse are frequently denied but with any abdominal crisis of undertermined aetiology physical abuse should be considered as a possible cause. A wide range of clinical presentations of abdominal injuries have been reported: ruptured spleen, kidney and liver, small and large bowel injuries, acute pancreatitis and damage to blood vessels.

Mrazek D, Mrazek M 1985 Child maltreatment. In: Rutter M, Hersov L (eds) Child and Adolescent Psychiatry, Modern Approaches, 2nd edn. Blackwell, Oxford

Smith S, Kunjukrishnan R 1985 Child abuse, perspectives on treatment and research. In: The Psychiatric Clinics of North America. Child Psychiatry December 1985. Saunders, Philadelphia

187 An illusion is a distortion of a real perception and it can be a normal phenomenon or a symptom of a functional disorder or a delirious state. Fright-

ened or anxious people may misidentify shadows, or creaking noises and attribute a sinister significance to them. In delirious states, such as delirium tremens, illusions frequently have a terrifying effect. Pareidolia is a type of illusion in which vivid illusions occur without any conscious effort on the part of the individual, such as those that occur when staring into a fire. Illusions must be distinguished from hallucinations and functional hallucinations. Whereas illusions are distortions of real perceptions, hallucinations are perceptions without an external stimulus. Illusions are generally a more transient phenomena than hallucinations. Functional hallucinations are hallucinations which occur simultaneously and in association with a real perception.

Hamilton M 1984 (ed) Fish's clinical psychopathology, 3rd edn. Wright, Bristol
Mullen P E 1986 The mental state and states of mind. In: Hill P, Murray R, Thorley A (eds) Essentials of Postgraduate Psychiatry 2nd edn. Grune and Stratton, London

188 This is a screening test performed on capillary blood during the neonatal period to detect raised levels of blood phenylalanine. The test depends on the ability of phenylalanine to promote the growth of Bacillus Subtilis in the presence of an inhibiting substance in a culture medium. The size of the growth is directly related to the amount of phenylalanine present thus enabling an accurate quantitative estimation to be made. The test is carried out on filter paper impregnated with blood from a heel prick sample taken between the ages of five and fourteen days. Earlier testing may give misleading levels in females. Infants homozygous for the phenylketonuria trait are not brain damaged at birth and will only become so if levels of phenylalanine are too high. Mental impairment is prevented in these children if a restricted phenylalanine diet is given and the serum levels of phenylalanine are maintained between 2.5 and 10 mg. per 100 mls.

Heaton–Ward W, Wiley Y 1984 Mental Handicap, 5th edn. Wright, Bristol

189 In England and Wales the crude suicide rate for men is approximately 9.7 per 100,000 and 6.2 per 100,000 for women. Statistics in 1975 showed a

gradual decline in suicide during the 1960s and continuing into the early 1970s. In England and Wales the overall fall in the rate during the 1960s was 34%. This decline was due principally to a decrease in suicide in the older age group—both males and females. There was relatively little change in the rate for the under 35 age group. In 1961 suicide in the elderly was 7–8 times more common than in young adults, compared with 3–4 times in 1974. However, in the period 1975–'80 the suicide rate has increased annually and this trend appears to be still continuing. In the period 1975–'80 there was an overall increase of 17%, the increase for males was 21% and 12% for females. The suicide rate for males increased in all age groups. The most alarming increases were in the age group 25–34 and 35–44 which showed an increase of 24% and 36% respectively. The age groups 75–84 also showed a 22% rate increase. In the USA and in most European countries suicide rates in age group 15–24 have shown a substantial increase with suicide being the third leading cause of death among adolescents in the USA. In England and Wales the suicide rate for age group 15–19 has increased since the 1950s for both males and females, with a substantial rise in males. While suicide is rare under 14 years, a small increase in female suicides in this age range has been reported.

Adelstein A, Mardon C 1975 Suicides, 1961–1974. In: Population Trends 2. Her Majesty's Stationery Office, London

McClure G M G 1984 Trends in suicide rates for England and Wales, 1975–1980. British Journal of Psychiatry 144: 119–126

McClure G M G 1984 Recent trends in suicide amongst the young. British Journal of Psychiatry 144: 134–138

190 This is a short acting drug that causes physiological arousal and euphoria. Its strong central nervous system stimulant effect produces increased wakefulness, confidence, hyperactivity and increased energy. It suppresses appetite and has peripheral sympathomimetic effects. A paranoid psychosis may be induced with hallucinations which may be auditory, visual or tactile. The tactile hallucinations produce the characteristic sensation of formication—of 'cocaine bugs' crawling under the skin. Depression and apathy are well defined features of abstinence and while

tolerance and psychological dependence may be severe, physical dependence does not occur. Cocaine is usually sniffed or 'snorted' and chronic snorting produces nasal membrane damage. When smoked there is an increased frequency of toxic effects.

Thorley A 1986 Drug problems. In: Hill P, Murray R, Thorley A (eds) Essentials of Postgraduate Psychiatry 2nd edn. Grune and Stratton, London

191 Family studies indicate that the morbid risk for bipolar and unipolar disorders is increased for the first degree relatives of those with bipolar manic-depression. While the rate varies from 10 to 40% between different surveys, the average morbidity risk is about 19% compared to a life time prevalence rate in the general population of 2.4%. Twin studies show that the concordance rate for bipolar disorders is between 70 and 80% for monozygotic twins and about 20% for dizygotic pairs. Price found on reviewing twelve cases of monozygotic twins, reared apart and where the index twin had an affective disorder, that there was a 67% concordance for affective disorder. Adoption studies indicate a higher rate for affective disorder among the biological as compared to the adoptive parents of probands with an affective disorder and one investigation reported that the morbidity risk for the biological parents was 2.5 times greater than that for the adoptive parents.

Bertelsen A, Harvald B, Hauge M 1977. A Danish twin study of manic-depressive disorders. British Journal of Psychiatry 130: 330–351
Mendlewicz J, Rainer J D 1977 Adoption study supporting genetic transmission in manic-depressive illness. Nature 268: 327–329
Nurnberger J I, Gershon E S 1982 Genetics. In: Paykel E S (ed) Handbook of Affective Disorders. Churchill Livingstone, Edinburgh

192 Approximately one-third of patients with Parkinsonism have cognitive deficits and while it was once thought that this was only associated with arteriosclerotic Parkinson's, more recent surveys have shown that it occurs with equal frequency in the idiopathic variety. Psychometric assessment tends to show that non-verbal ability is more affected than verbal scores on intelligence subtests and that the degree of cognitive impairment is not wholly related to either the severity of the disease

or the degree of depression which can accompany it.

Lishman W A 1978 Other disorders affecting the nervous system. In: Organic Psychiatry. Blackwell, London

Mindham R H S 1970 Psychiatric Symptoms in Parkinsonism. Journal of Neurology, Neurosurgery and Psychiatry 33: 188–191

193 The main effect is that of impairment of recent memory. While immediate memory, such as is tested with digit span retention, is intact, as soon as the patient is attending to further information the former is lost. This results in an inability to memorise current events and in disorientation in time. Retrograde amnesia is also a feature and often covers a period of months to years before the lesion. There is a disorder of time sense and as a result most events will be recalled in a disordered way and often as if they had occurred recently. In pure diencephalic lesions distant memory beyond the retrograde period is intact and intellect and behaviour is unaffected. In Korsakoff's psychosis, the disorder most frequently associated with diencephalic damage, cognitive function and affect are disturbed since the pathological lesions are not confined to the mammillary bodies and thalamic nuclei.

Lishman W A 1978 Symptoms and syndromes with regional affiliations. In: Organic Psychiatry. Blackwell, Oxford

194 A favourable outcome is associated with an acute onset, short episode, precipitating life event, prominent affective symptoms and no previous psychiatric history. A normal premorbid personality, with good work record and social relationships and a satisfactory psychosexual adjustment indicates a more favourable outcome as does a family history of affective illness, negative family history of schizophrenia and older age at onset. Women have a slightly better prognosis than men and marriage appears to have a protective role against further relapse. Poor prognostic factors include low IQ, low social class, chronicity, early age of onset, lack of insight, blunting of affect, poor premorbid personality and a positive family history. Thought disorder, hallucinations and delusions do not have any prognostic value.

British Medical Journal 1977 (Editorial) First attacks
of schizophrenia. British Medical Journal (i)
733–734
Murray R 1979 Schizophrenia. In: Hill P, Murray R,
Thorley A (eds) Essentials of Postgraduate
Psychiatry. Academic Press, London

195 This term is applied to those children whose
reading ability falls two standard errors below the
mean level that their age, schooling and IQ would
predict. In the Isle of Wight epidemiological
study, the prevalence was 4% while in inner
London the rate was 10%. The aetiology is uncertain with biological, developmental, social,
cultural and neurological factors all being implicated. It is encountered in children from all back-
grounds but is three times more common in boys
than in girls. The most common mode of presentation is for the 6 to 9 year old child to be found
lagging behind his peers in learning to read at
school. Delay in speech and language skills are
also associated. Writing and more particularly
spelling is markedly impaired. Clumsiness and
visuomotor difficulties are seen. A learning
disorder in arithmetic is commonly seen. Retarded
readers have a lower verbal IQ than performance
IQ on the Weschler Adult Intelligence Scale.
These children come from families which are large
and have a background of reading difficulties.
There is a marked association between reading
retardation and antisocial behaviour; in the Isle of
Wight study one-third of ten year old children
with reading retardation were diagnosed as having
conduct disorders and conversely one-third of
conduct disordered children were more than
twenty-eight months retarded in their reading
compared with the level predicted from the IQ.
Prognosis is generally poor with difficulties often
persisting into adult life. Even if reading is
improved, spelling difficulties commonly persist.

Russell G 1983 Learning disorders. In: Russell G,
Hersov L (eds) Handbook of Psychiatry 4 The
neuroses and personality disorders. Cambridge
University Press, Cambridge
Rutter M, Yule W 1975 The concept of specific
reading retardation. Journal of Child Psychology
16: 181–197
Rutter M, Tizard J, Yule M, Graham P, Whitmore K
1976 Isle of Wight Studies. 1964–74. Psychological
Medicine 6: 313–332

196 These support systems have formal and informal components. The formal components consist of the set of basic entitlements to some elderly people, such as widows' pensions, the statutory agencies that operate the economic and social policies of the Government and the semi-formal organisations such as church groups. These groups possess technical expertise and resources. The informal network consist of the extended family, neighbours and friends who offer the main support for the generality of the elderly. They are more available to the elderly for unpredictable events, are familiar with the particular individual and the situation and can assist with the daily tasks of living and provide support during times of illness.

Levy R, Post F 1982 (eds) The psychiatry of late life. Blackwell, Oxford

197 Crow suggests that there may be two main sub-types within the concept of schizophrenia—Type I and Type II. Type I is closely associated with positive symptoms such as hallucinations and delusions while Type II is associated with features of the defect state: social withdrawal, reduced motivation, flattening of affect and intellectual deterioration. Type I is characterised by a fairly acute course, good response to neuroleptic medication and absence of intellectual impairment. Computerised tomography is generally normal and there is a positive family history. Type II shows a chronic deterioration, has a poor response to neuroleptics, may show cognitive impairment on psychological testing and seems to be associated with enlarged cerebral ventricles. Pathologically Type I is associated with an increase in dopamine activity while Type II involves a brain degenerative process of unknown aetiology, characterised by structural brain damage. Variations in prolactin concentrations and in follicle stimulating and luteinizing hormones are postulated to be related to the dopaminergic over-activity assumed to underlie the positive symptoms component. Changes in growth hormone response to apomorphine is related to Type II and may correlate with structural changes.

Crow T J 1980 Molecular pathology of schizophrenia: More than one disease process? British Medical Journal 280: 66–68

Crow T J 1985 The two-syndrome concept: Origins
    and current concepts. Schizophrenia Bulletin
    11: 471–486

198 Delinquent behaviour is thought to arise through
an interaction between temperamental attributes,
individual characteristics and family and environmental influences. Individual characteristics most
frequently associated with antisocial behaviour are
cognitive and educational retardation. Rutter
noted a significant association with reading retardation and antisocial behaviour. However, it is
uncertain whether reading retardation leads to
antisocial behaviour or the converse holds. Boys
are more often affected. Delinquency in adolescence
has often been preceded by aggressive conduct in
early childhood. Other factors thought to be
implicated are hyperactivity and attentional deficits, autonomic reactivity and adverse temperamental factors. The family characteristics strongly
associated include parental criminality, ineffective
supervision and discipline, familial disharmony,
weak parent-child relationships, large families and
low socio-economic status. Research shows an
increased prevalence of antisocial behaviour in
particular schools. The factors involved in the
school influence seems to be related to the general
intellectual ability and social status of the pupils,
the school ethos and level of social organisation.
Urban areas show significantly higher rates than
rural ones and even within cities there are markedly varying rates of crime. There is some
evidence that in those children who are liable to
aggressive behaviour, antisocial acts may be
provoked by television violence and other media
influences.

Hill P 1986 The psychiatry of adolescence. In: Hill P,
    Murray R, Thorley A (eds) Essentials of
    Postgraduate Psychiatry 2nd edn. Grune and
    Stratton, London
Rutter M, Giller H 1983 (eds) Juvenile delinquency.
    Trends and perspectives. Penguin, London

199 Assessment should take into account both
biological and psychological aspects of the
complaint. The first step is to consider the nature
and developmental history of the impotence in
order to determine whether it is of sudden onset,
occurs selectively or whether spontaneous,
masturbatory or morning erections continue to

occur. The frequency of attempted sexual inter-course, both past and in the present, masturba-tory activity and fantasies, both past and present, sexual experience including homosexual experi-ence, extent of sexual knowledge and technique used and contraceptive methods used should all be discussed. The relationship with the sexual partner, their patterns of behaviour with each other and the partner's attitude to sexual activity should be determined. Environmental conditions should be enquired about, such as sharing bedrooms and home stresses. The family and past personal history should take account of the patient's background, upbringing, childhood, traumas such as incest, sex education and the family's attitude to sex. The patient's mental state is assessed as depression and excessive anxiety can be associated with impotence. The patient's medical history should be examined for evidence of the numerous cardiovascular, haematological, endocrinological, neurological, genito-urinary and pharmacological conditions that are associated with impotence and a full general physical exam-ination should be performed. Biochemical screening, hormonal assays or measurement of nocturnal penile tumescence may be indicated following the clinical assessment. Where possible the patient and his partner should be seen together to explore their attitudes to the problem, their levels of commitment to each other and to discern whether there is sufficient motivation and resources for change.

Kaplan H S 1978 The new sex therapy. Ballière Tindall and Peregrine Books, London
Karacan I, Salis P 1980 Diagnosis and treatment of erectile impotence. In: The Psychiatric Clinics of North America April: 97–113 Saunders, Philadelphia

200 The results of a study by Hsu in 1980 and by Schwartz and Thompson in 1981, which typify what other large scale studies had found, indicate that two-thirds of anorexics will be at near normal weight several years after treatment. In terms of weight and disturbed eating habits, these studies found that 49% had recovered completely, 31% showed some improvement and 18% remained unchanged. Regular menstruation was reported to have been restored in about 50% of the cases in most studies. The mortality rate varies from 0% to 25% but both reviews arrived at a typical

mortality of 6%. The causes of death include suicide, electrolyte imbalance and gross inanition. In terms of psychiatric status and psychological functioning up to two-thirds of patients were still preoccupied with weight and body shape despite a normal weight. Many led isolated lives and experienced relationship difficulties and depressive and obsessional symptoms were common at follow-up.

Hsu L K G 1980 Outcome of anorexia nervosa. A review of the literature, (1954–1978). Archives of General Psychiatry 37: 1041–1046

Schwartz D, Thompson M G 1981 Do anorexics get well? Current research and future trends. American Journal of Psychiatry 138: 319–323

201 The conventional electrode placement is the bifrontotemporal position: 4 cms above the midpoint of a line drawn from the lateral angle of the eye to the external auditory meatus.

Freeman C P L 1979 Electroconvulsive therapy: its current clinical use. British Journal of Hospital Medicine 21: 281–292

202 Personal, religious, cultural, familial and other factors can alter the response to grief. Childhood experiences, especially loss of significant persons and responses to past bereavement may be important. Personality factors in the bereaved person, psychiatric and physical illness will modify the response. The type of death, whether sudden or expected, the management of the dying period and the characteristics of the relationship between the deceased and the surviving person may all be factors which affect the expression of grief. Age and sex, both of the deceased and the survivor, are also relevant. The expression of grief is altered by religious and cultural tradition. Other factors which may alter the response include the presence or absence of secondary stresses at the time of bereavement, such as loss of income, change of home or difficulties with children, lack of social and family supports, unemployment and having dependent children.

Parkes C 1972 Bereavement. Studies of grief in adult life. Penguin, London

203 It is a self-administered 48 item personality questionnaire which measures two major factors:

extraversion–introversion and neuroticism. Eysenck factor analysed responses from large groups of psychiatric patients and normal subjects and found that many of the personality differences could be summarised in terms of their differences along two main independent dimensions: introversion–extraversion and neuroticism. He claims that those who score high on neuroticism are liable to neurotic disorders and those who are introverted develop dysthymic disorders. A vast amount of research has attempted to put the personality dimensions on a firmer biological footing by producing evidence of their genetic and psychobiological links. The inventory also incorporates a 'Lie Scale' which enables the tester to assess the extent to which the subject responded in a socially desirable manner. A more recent development of the questionnaire includes a scale for measuring a third factor of personality called 'psychotism' which seems to be more akin to psychopathy.

Mann A, Murray R 1986 Measurement in Psychiatry. In: Hill P, Murray R, Thorley A (eds) Essentials of Postgraduate Psychiatry 2nd edn. Grune and Stratton, London

204 The use of ECT in schizophrenia has declined over the years as neuroleptics have become the treatment of first choice and as the disorder has become more clearly defined to exclude affective psychotic states. While most of the earlier research in this area is of limited value because of the absence of well defined diagnostic criteria, a number of pointers have emerged. ECT has been shown to be particularly effective in catatonic schizophrenia, but there is now some doubt whether the catatonic features belong to the schizophrenic category or whether it is a type of affective disorder and thus should be considered as schizo-affective disorder. Taylor, (1981) found in a double blind trial of schizophrenics who were on neuroleptics that those given ECT showed a significantly better response than those receiving anaesthesia and a subconvulsive current. Those with affective symptoms, paranoid delusions, auditory hallucinations and delusions of passivity showed the best response.

Fraser M 1982 ECT in other conditions— schizophrenia. In: ECT—a clinical guide. Wiley, Chichester

Taylor P 1981 ECT: The preliminary report of a trial
in schizophrenic patients. In: Palmer R L (ed)
Electroconvulsive Therapy: An appraisal. Oxford
University Press, Oxford

205 Details about awareness, orientation, attentiveness, ability to concentrate and recall events, level
of general information about current events and
an account of academic and employment records
will usually provide a reliable estimate of cognitive
function. Orientation is checked by asking the
patient his name, the day, date, month and year,
to approximate the time of day and to state his
address and current whereabouts. Ability to
concentrate can be tested by asking him to
subtract serial sevens from 100, repeat digits in
correct and reverse order and by generally
observing his attentiveness during the interview.
Immediate and recent memory is assessed by
getting the patient to recall digits or addresses and
a sentence immediately and after 3–5 minutes
when he has been attending to other information.
A disorder of remote memory will usually be
evident when the account of sequence of events
in the patient's life is inconsistent or does not tally
with information obtained from a relative. The
patient's grasp of general information about
current events is checked by enquiring about
items of local and national interest, such as heads
of government and public personalities. A
disparity between the academic or employment
record and his present status and interests or
ability to cope with items during the interview
may be significant. Simple tests of intelligence
such as the Mill Hill Vocabulary test or Raven's
Progressive Matrices may be employed as an
addendum to the mental state examination.

Departmental Teaching Committee of the Institute of
Psychiatry 1973 Notes on eliciting and recording
clinical information. Oxford University Press,
Oxford

206 Cannabis is the generic name for various preparations of cannabis sativa or hemp plant and it
is grown commercially both for its fibre content
and for use as an illicit drug with psychological
effects. Psycho-active substances are present in all
parts of the plant, but they are found in highest
concentrations in the flowering tops and leaves of
the plant. Both the dried leaves, marijuana and

the resin, hashish, have been used for centuries. Concentrated extracts in the form of hash oil are also prepared. The foremost active ingredient is tetrahydro-cannabinol. The percentage concentration of tetrahydro-cannabinol varies greatly ranging from 0–4% in American herbal preparations to between 5–15% in Asian resinous material. In the USA some two-thirds of young adults report having taken marijuana and one-third report current use. Prevalence studies in Britain range from rates of 2% to 40% with about 10% of young people emerging as having tried cannabis at some time.

Fishburne P M, Cisin I 1980 National survey on drug abuse. Main findings 1979. National Institute of Drug Abuse (NIDA). Rockville, Maryland
Granville–Grossman K 1979 Psychiatric aspects of cannabis use. In: Granville–Grossman K (ed) Recent Advances in Clinical Psychiatry. Churchill Livingstone, Edinburgh

207   The patient experiences his thoughts, feelings or actions as being foreign and controlled against his will by some outside influence. He may attribute this experience to hypnosis, radio waves, machines or other controlling agents. Schneider claimed that these experiences, termed passivity phenomena, are diagnostic of schizophrenia in the absence of coarse brain disease. Thought insertion, thought withdrawal and thought broadcast are passivity phenomena. Thought insertion is the experience that outside alien thoughts are being imposed on the patient; thought withdrawal is the experience that his own thoughts have been taken away from him and thought broadcast is the experience that his thoughts have been passively diffused or lost to the outside world against his will. Made impulses, acts and feelings describe the experience of actions being under external control. With somatic passivity phenomenon, the patient actually experiences bodily sensations as being produced by an outside agency. Much confusion among Anglo-American investigators revolves around the exact boundaries of these phenomenon: whether just the control is lost or whether the thoughts, emotions and actions have taken on an alien quality as well as being under outside influence.

Koehler K 1979 First rank symptoms of schizophrénia. Questions concerning clinical

boundaries. British Journal of Psychiatry
134: 236–248

Mellor C S 1970 First rank symptoms of
schizophrenia. British Journal of Psychiatry
117: 15–23

208 Rutter notes that adolescent disorders tend to run
true to type in that marked symptom variability
is not a feature of adolescent morbidity. Antisocial
disorders, for instance, in late adolescence are
found almost exclusively in those who have
previously had a conduct disorder. Similarly,
emotionally disordered adolescents, if they
continue to show disturbance, will present with
neurotic problems. A few of these may in fact
develop psychoses. The prognosis for psychoses
in adolescence is not dissimilar from the outlook
when the onset is in early adulthood. Emotional
disorders have the most favourable outcome with
83% improving and about half of those with
conduct disorder improve. Thus psychiatric
disorder needs to be taken just as seriously when
it occurs in adolescence as at any other age.

Rutter M (ed) 1979 Changing youth in a changing
society. Patterns of adolescent development and
disorder. Nuffield Provincial Hospital Trust,
London

209 Depression is the most common psychiatric
disorder in Parkinson's syndrome. Varying
degrees of depressive features have been noted in
30 to 90% of those with this syndrome, while
mania is a rare occurrence. The depression is
often reactive in nature and related to the physical
limitations of the condition and its implications
for the patient's future. A significant correlation
has been found between the main physical symptoms of Parkinson's and the severity of depression
and the therapeutic response of both to L-dopa
was noted to be comparable. However, many clinicians are impressed by the high frequency of
depression in this disorder compared to more
disabling conditions, its tendency to respond to antidepressant medication, and it having a course
which is independent of the physical symptoms
and the fact that occasionally depressive symptoms predate the physical features.

Lishman W A 1978 Other disorders affecting the
nervous system. In: Organic Psychiatry. Blackwell,
Oxford

Mindham R H S 1974 Psychiatric aspects of
Parkinson's disease. British Journal of Hospital
Medicine 11: 411–414

210 The aetiology of tardive dyskinesia is unknown.
Epidemiological studies suggest a strong association between use of neuroleptic medication and
development of the syndrome, but it is not
confined to people on long term neuroleptics.
Drug discontinuation leads to an exacerbation of
the dyskinesia and increasing the dose gives
temporary relief. Anticholinergics can uncover
latent tardive dyskinesia or exacerbate existing
symptoms. An increase in the sensitivity of the
post-synaptic dopamine receptors in the corpus
striatum has been implicated as part of the causal
pathway. Other explanations include an imbalance
between dopaminergic and cholinergic transmitter
functions and an alteration in the concentration
of gamma-aminobutyric acid. Drugs which affect
these systems have all been used to treat the
syndrome with varying success. Increasing the
dose of the antipsychotic drug has short term
gains but its use is not advocated. Tetrabenazine
has shown some superiority over placebo. Other
drugs which have been recommended include
benzodiazepines, reserpine, choline, physostigmine, lecithin, sodium valporate, baclofen and
gamma-methylparatyrosine. A large number of
other treatments have also been claimed to be
useful but they have not been properly evaluated.
Although there are a large number of reports
concerning drug treatment of tardive dyskinesia,
most cause only slight to moderate improvement
in fewer than half of the patients treated. The
most effective technique is early detection with
dosage reduction or discontinuation of the neuroleptic. However, prevention is all important and
strict guidelines regarding use of neuroleptics
should be adhered to.

Klawaus H L, Goetz C G, Perlik S 1980 Tardive
dyskinesia: Review and update. American Journal of
Psychiatry 137
McKay A, Sheppard G 1986 Pharmacotherapeutic
trials in tardive dyskinesia. In: Kerr A, Snaith P
(eds) Contemporary Issues in Schizophrenia. Gaskell
Psychiatry Series

211 Enuresis is more common among males and tends
to run in families. Some 70% of enuretics have a

first degree relative who wets the bed and twin studies show that monozygotic twins display a significantly higher degree of concordance than dizygotic pairs. Approximately 5% of enuretics have urinary tract infections and physical abnormalities such as small bladder capacity and immature configuration of the vesical base plate are only rarely encountered. Low socio-economic status, large families with much disruption and parental delinquency and institutional upbringing are all associated with increased rates of enuresis. In a small number of enuretics the incontinence relates to mental retardation, neurological anomalies or encopresis. Children who experience stressful life events at age 3 to 4 years have a two-fold increased risk of developing enuresis. Such events include divorce, admissions to hospital, family disruption or birth of a sibling. Enuretic children, particularly girls, show a significantly increased prevalence of psychiatric morbidity, but such disturbances are only present in a minority. No specific psychopathological picture emerges. Psychiatric problems tend to be more common in children who wet by day as well as by night.

Kolvin I, MacKeith R C, Meadow S R 1973 (eds) Bladder control and enuresis. Clinical Development Medicine 48–49. SIMP/Heinemann, London
Taylor E 1983 Disturbances of toilet function. In: Russell G, Hersov L (eds) Handbook of Psychiatry 4. The neuroses and personality disorders. Cambridge University Press, Cambridge

212 This is characterised by a stepwise deterioration in memory and intellect, focal neurological signs and evidence of cardiovascular disease. Men are more commonly affected. Evidence of arteriosclerosis may be seen in peripheral arterial vessels and hypertension is a frequent feature. Abrupt episodes may occur with features of hemiparesis, dysphasia, dysarthria and visual difficulties. Somatic complaints are common and epileptic seizures occur in 25% of cases. Other physical findings may include pseudobulbar palsy, Parkinson's disease, extensor plantar and abnormal tendon reflexes. The mental state fluctuates frequently and onset of nocturnal confusional episodes is a characteristic feature. Personality is relatively well preserved until late and the retention of insight may cause profound depression. Lability of mood is common and there is a tend-

ency towards explosive emotional outbursts. The course of the illness is characteristically intermittent with abrupt exacerbations and occasionally periods of remission. Each episode is generally followed by an increase in severity of the dementia. Death is attributable to ischaemic heart disease in approximately 50% of cases while others succumb to cerebral infarction or renal complications.

Gurland B, Birkett D 1983 The senile and presenile dementias. In: Lader M (ed) Handbook of Psychiatry 2. Mental disorders and somatic illness. Cambridge University Press, Cambridge

213 Several different psychodynamic views of depression have been developed over the years, most of which are an extension of Freud's original explanation. In his paper 'Mourning and Melancholia' he drew attention to the resemblance between grief and depression, noting that in the latter the loss was more symbolic than real. He suggested that following a loss the lost object is dealt with by incorporation into the self and the self and object are bitterly attacked, or as he later elaborated, condemned by the superego. Rado restated the early psychoanalytic views and he saw the depressive as somebody who was in great need of narcissistic supplies to bolster his frail self-esteem and this was associated with extreme unconscious anger because of the dependence on others. In the 1950s the ego psychology view was developed by Bibring and others. They proposed that depression emerged from a sense of helplessness felt by the ego when it became aware of its inability to attain its ideals. The 1970s saw the emergence of the Kleinian view of depression based on traumatic infantile events and the quality of the mother-child relationship. She developed the concept that children who are insecure in being loved do not internalize good 'objects' and are predisposed to the depressive position in later life.

Checkley S 1986 Affective disorder: Depression. In: Hill P, Murray R, Thorley A (eds) Essentials of Postgraduate Psychiatry 2nd edn. Grune and Stratton, London
Mendelson M 1982 The psychodynamics of depression. In: Paykel E S (ed) Handbook of Affective Disorders. Churchill Livingstone, Edinburgh

214 The initial home assessment is seen as essential by many psychogeriatricians and should preferably be made by the consultant with one or two members of the team. In the home environment the patient is usually at his optimum and moving a confused old person to a hospital setting often worsens the confusion and presents him in a poor light. The patient's personality and past and present lifestyle is often visually expressed by the manner in which he keeps his home and by his behaviour within it. The physical environment can be observed, its amenities or lack of them and its potential risks, such as rickety stairs, can be seen at first hand. Other clues may be the absence of food or the presence of the incontinent sheets or an accumulation of bottles. The visit enables one to meet those who provide social support such as family and neighbours and a comprehensive collateral history can be obtained. One can also assess the resources, financial and social, which may help if eventual resettlement is required.

Williamson A 1981 Evaluation of home visiting of patients by physician in geriatric medicine. British Medical Journal 282: 718–720

215 The interviewer must develop a sympathetic and empathetic relationship with the patient's feelings. This is best done by listening to the patient's account, by not asking very direct questions about the delusions, by not attempting to refute his ideas and by concentrating on the level of his upset feelings. These interviewing techniques will usually encourage patients to speak more openly about their delusions and with the occasional tactful question the strength of their beliefs and whether they are likely to act upon them can be assessed. The interview should be conducted in an open area where the patient and the interviewer will feel more comfortable with other staff in the vicinity. It is inadvisable to agree with the patient's delusions as this deceit will in turn lead to further mistrust. If you consider that the patient needs admission to hospital it is prudent to make arrangements without him knowing about them. When the plans are finalised the patient should be told in the presence of nursing personnel that they are being admitted to hospital immediately. This avoids unnecessary arguments during which the patient might flee

from the emergency room and is the safest approach for patient and staff.

Perry S W 1984 Management of functional psychoses. In: Dubin W R, Hanke N, Nickens H W (eds) Psychiatric Emergencies. Churchill Livingstone Inc, New York

216 The technique is a form of aversive therapy based entirely on the use of a patient's imagery or fantasies. The patient imagines a highly unpleasant or disgusting scene and associates this repeatedly with mental images connected with his deviant behaviour. The procedure has advantages over aversive therapy in that it is less unpleasant, is simpler to implement and can be used easily by the patient. It has been used to treat a wide range of sexual deviations often in combination with other techniques. Its value has still to be proven.

Peck D F, McGuire R J 1988 Behavioural and cognitive therapies. In: Kendell R E, Zealley A K (eds) Companion to Psychiatric Studies, 4th edn. Churchill Livingstone, Edinburgh

217 A wide range of functional and organic disorders can produce stupor but in a psychiatric setting most will be functional and can be distinguished from other causes. A past history of psychiatric illness, the manner of onset of the stupor, the type of facial expression and an ability to recall events occurring in the environment during the stupor will help to identify those of functional origin. Particular attention must be paid to the neurological examination and to the exclusion of diencephalic and brain stem lesions. In schizophrenia the stupor is mainly that of a catatonic state and the features of this syndrome, including the patient's facial expression, will usually indicate the diagnosis. Depressive stupor is a form of extreme psychomotor retardation in which the diagnosis will be apparent from the patient's dejected apathetic appearance and reduced eye movements. Manic stupor results from extreme mental hyperactivity and this is often reflected in rapid eye movements. Hysterical or psychogenic stupor is usually stress related, tends to wax and wane and the patient is likely to show a response if they are in an uncomfortable position or when an emotionally important topic is discussed. Signs of conversion hysteria are usually present. An interview

conducted during a slow intravenous injection of
sodium amytal will often help to confirm those of
functional origin by giving access to the patient's
thought content.

Lishman W A 1978 Differential diagnosis. In: Organic
    Psychiatry. Blackwell, Oxford

218 Neurosyphilitic disorders rarely figure in present
day psychiatry. Dementia is probably the most
common mode of presentation of General Paresis
of the Insane (GPI). It starts insidiously and is
often preceded by personality or mood disturbances before the cognitive disturbance is evident.
Minor changes in temperament with moodiness,
apathy, temper tantrums and emotional lability
are often noted in retrospect to have been present
for a number of months beforehand and these
reflect frontal lobe damage. The cognitive disturbance is usually evident as episodic forgetfulness,
difficulty with calculations, poor concentration,
eventually proceeding to a full blown dementia.
Another manifestation of GPI, probably occurring
with equal frequency, is the depressive form.
While the quality of the depressive affect may be
shallow and the symptoms tend to be relieved by
environmental factors, GPI can present as a
typical delusional depression indistinguishable
from the functional variety. Other forms such as
the taboparietic and grandiose types are extremely
rare, but these and other forms can mimic schizophreniform states and mania.

Dewhurst K 1969 The neurosyphilitic psychoses
    today: a survey of 91 cases. British Journal of
    Psychiatry 115: 31–38
Luxon L, Lees A J, Greenwood R J 1979
    Neurosyphilis today. Lancet 1: 90–93

219 This is a disorder where the skin lesions are self
induced. The lesions are destructive, bizarre,
often necrotic and asymmetrical and do not
conform in their appearances to those which occur
in natural skin disorders. Dermatitis artefacta is
more commonly encountered in young single
women. Sneddon and Sneddon reviewed forty-
three patients some of whom continued to
produce lesions for several years. A wide variety
of psychiatric illnesses, personality problems and
social difficulties were described. The authors
concluded that the prognosis was relatively poor
and seemed more related to a process of matu-

ration and changing circumstances rather than any
specific therapeutic measure.

Russell G 1983 Skin disorders and dermatitis artefacta.
In: Russell G, Hersov L (eds) Handbook of
Psychiatry 4 The neuroses and personality disorders.
Cambridge University Press, Cambridge
Sneddon I, Sneddon J 1975 Self-inflicted injury: A
follow up study of 43 patients. British Medical
Journal 3: 527–530

220 Memory impairment is the major side effect associated with ECT. There is a short and rapidly
dwindling retrograde amnesia, a post ECT confusional period lasting 20–40 minutes and a longer
anterograde amnesia reflected by a reduced ability
to retain new information in the twenty-four hours
following ECT. Nominal aphasia is probably quite
common, but is often only remarked upon by the
more obsessional patients who also seem to be
more prone to depersonalisation following the
treatment. Headache in the hours after treatment
is not uncommon and it responds promptly to
minor analgesics. Mania may also be induced by
ECT and it is more likely to occur in those with
either a personal or family history of bipolar
affective disorder. The mortality rate associated
with ECT has been calculated as one in every
28,000 treatments, but this figure will obviously
be affected by the physical status of the sample.
Coronary thrombosis, cerebral haemorrhage and
pulmonary embolism are the main causes of
death. Non-fatal complications include disloca-
tions, fractures, fat embolism and perforation of,
or bleeding from, a peptic ulcer.

Squire L R, Slater P C, Miller P L 1981. Retrograde
amnesia and bilateral electroconvulsive therapy.
Archives of General Psychiatry 38: 89–95
Weeks D, Freeman C P L, Kendell R E 1981 Does
ECT produce enduring cognitive deficits. In: Palmer
R L (ed) Electroconvulsive therapy: An appraisal.
Oxford University Press, Oxford

221 It is a self-administered 60 item questionnaire
designed to detect non-psychotic psychiatric
morbidity of recent onset in general practice. It
enquires about the appearance of new distressing
symptoms and about one's ability to cope with
daily activity. The questions form the 'lowest
common multiple' of symptoms encountered in
various mental disorders and as a non-specific
indicator of psychiatric morbidity it is equivalent

to the ESR in general medicine. There are four subscales: somatic symptoms, anxiety and insomnia, social dysfunction and severe depression. It has been shown to be both specific and sensitive in its detection of psychiatric symptoms and high scores indicate the likelihood of the subject being a psychiatric case, but it will not indicate the diagnosis. Shortened versions of the questionnaire are now available. It is also used as a research case screening instrument.

Goldberg D P, Blackwell B 1970 Psychiatric illness in general practice: A detailed study using a new method of case identification. British Medical Journal 2: 439–443

222 The incidence of alcoholism in females has increased dramatically in the past decade in the UK. The ratio of men to women admitted to hospital with alcohol problems fell from 3.9:1 in 1964 to 2.7:1 in 1975. Female drinkers admit to a greater appreciation of the psychological effect of alcohol and show less enjoyment of the drinking process itself. Women alcoholics often follow a 'telescoped' course with a more rapid deterioration than males and up to 50% of them drink alone. They show more alcohol related disorders than males in that they have an increased susceptibility to liver cirrhosis and are more likely to develop Wernicke–Korsakoff's syndrome. Compared with men they show more mental problems, have more personal crises and are more likely to attempt suicide. There is a higher rate of alcoholism among the first degree relatives of female alcoholics than there is among the relatives of their male counterparts.

Camberwell Council on Alcoholism 1980 Women and alcohol. Tavistock, London
Saunders J B, Davis M, Williams R 1981 Do women develop alcoholic liver disease more readily than men? British Journal of Medicine 282: 1140–1143

223 While child sexual abuse is not at all confined to lower socio-economic groups, the evidence suggests that children from poorer families are at somewhat higher risk. American figures also suggest that social isolation and households where the mother is the only head of the household are vulnerability factors. Girls are more often abused sexually and for both sexes, late childhood and early adolescence are relatively peak periods for

sexual abuse. The numbers of children under five who come to the attention of concerned agencies is apparently rising steadily and even infants are affected. Though not yet empirically established, it is frequently reported how female victims of sexual abuse appear to have taken on a 'wife and mother' type role and that they may tend to be attention seeking. As Mrazek and Mrazek say however, the child's role as a participating victim has yet to be fully understood.

Mrazek D, Mrazek M 1985 Child maltreatment. In: Rutter M, Hersov L (eds) Child and Adolescent Psychiatry Modern Approaches, 2nd edn. Blackwell, Oxford

Smith S, Kunjukrishnan R 1985 Child abuse, perspectives on treatment and research. In: The Psychiatric Clinics of North America. Child Psychiatry. December 1985 Saunders, Philadelphia

224   The onset of the condition is usually insidious, with dieting and increased exercise. Gradually in their 'pursuit of thinness' patients with anorexia nervosa avoid, particularly, carbohydrates and fats, may induce vomiting, exercise excessively and may abuse purgatives, diuretics and appetite suppressants. In approximately 50% of instances pathological dieting is punctuated by episodes of binge eating. After binging they generally induce vomiting, are full of remorse and guilt, which further intensifies their efforts to lose weight. Regular weighing, sometimes hourly, becomes part of the ritual. Despite apparent food refusal, their appetite persists and they are intensely preoccupied with food and often enjoy cooking elaborate meals for others. Some 10% to 20% admit to stealing food. Body image disturbance is frequently present but is not pathonomonic. Other symptoms include increased sensitivity to cold, constipation, decreased libido, depression, impaired concentration, fatigue and insomnia. Amenorrhoea in the female and loss of libido in the male are usual diagnostic criteria, yet regular menstruation may persist in some patients. The mean age of onset is 17 years and females with this disorder are predominantly from socio-economic class I. Approximately one-third had been overweight premorbidly. Marked weight loss is apparent and subcutaneous fat is reduced. Axillary and pubic hair is present, there is no breast atrophy and lanugo hair covers the cheeks, arms and back. Blood pressure is usually de-

creased and bradycardia, hypothermia and peripheral cyanosis are evident. Both self-induced vomiting and purgative abuse may precipitate tetany, peripheral paraesthesia, dehydration, muscle weakness and loss of energy. The patient may also have dental erosion, a chronic hoarse voice, parotid enlargement, finger clubbing, abdominal pain and steatorrhoea.

Russell G 1983 Anorexia nervosa and bulimia nervosa. In: Russell G, Hersov L (eds) Handbook of Psychiatry 4 The neuroses and personality disorders. Cambridge University Press, Cambridge

225 The usual consequences quoted in the literature derive from case material only and nearly every psychological disorder has at some time been linked with sexual abuse. The major group of sequelae is in relation to sexual adjustment and includes precocious interest and preoccupation with sexual matters, increased masturbatory activity, despair regarding the inability to control sexual urges, promiscuity and molestation of younger children. As adults there may be an aversion to sexual activity, homosexuality, prostitution, involvement in other incestuous or abusing relationships and lack of protection of one's own children from sexual abuse. Most strikingly studies of teenage prostitute runaways and drug addicts suggest that 50% of these groups have been sexually abused. Nevertheless, not all victims suffer these effects. Protective and vulnerability factors are unknown and a methodologically sound prospective study of the consequences of child sexual abuse is needed.

Mrazek D, Mrazek M 1985 Child maltreatment. In: Rutter M, Hersov L (eds) Child and Adolescent Psychiatry Modern Approaches, 2nd edn. Blackwell, Oxford
Smith S, Kunjukrishnan R 1985 Child abuse, perspectives on treatment and research. In: The Psychiatric Clinics of North America Child Psychiatry, December, 1985. Saunders, Philadelphia

226 Insight or self-understanding is not a unitary concept. It occurs when the individual discovers something about himself, his behaviour, motivational system, fantasy life or his unconscious. Self-understanding is often considered to occur at two levels, an intellectual one in which the sense of knowing is evident and at an emotional level in which the feeling aspect is realised. Insight may

mean the degree of understanding that a patient has about his condition, his understanding of the underlying causation of the condition, his understanding of his own psychological processes, of the nature of his relationships with others and with his environment. Group therapists recognise two chief categories: interpersonal and psychogenetic insight. In interpersonal insight the individual gains understanding into what he is doing to himself and with other people while psychogenetic insight attempts to help people understand the origins of one's problems.

Lewis A 1934 The psychopathology of insight. British Journal of Medicine Psychology 14: 332

227 The principal features include a feeling of relaxation and euphoria. Short term memory and concentration are impaired, talk becomes circumlocutory and there is an enhancement and distortion of perceptions. Time sense is characteristically disturbed, often with remarkable lengthening of subjective appreciation of time spans. Sympathetic arousal is evident with tachycardia, dry mouth and tremor. Other physical signs include gastrointestinal disturbance, vasodilation, conjunctival reddening, diuresis and increased respiratory rate. The intensity and nature of experience induced by the drug varies greatly and depends on the naiviety of the subject, his expectations and the situation in which the drug is being taken. Occasionally, the subject may become very frightened and experience a sense of helplessness and loss of control and these may be associated with persecutory ideas. Intake of very large doses may result in malaise, hypotension, vomiting and ultimately coma, though this is very rare. A transient psychotic state which resolves within days of stopping the drug and is characterised by paranoid delusions and hallucinations occurring in clear consciousness, has been described. Tolerance appears to develop to the drug but the question of whether dependence occurs remains controversial.

Hamid Ghodse A 1983 Drug dependence and intoxication. In: Lader M (ed) Handbook of Psychiatry 2, Mental disorders and somatic illness. Cambridge University Press, Cambridge
Thorley A 1986 Drug problems. In: Hill P, Murray R, Thorley A (eds) Essentials of Postgraduate Psychiatry, 2nd edn. Grune and Stratton, London

228   It would be important at the outset to establish as far as possible whether the depression is part of a life long pattern, or due to the physical, neurological or cognitive deficits following the stroke. Not infrequently minor deficits such as defective comprehension, apraxia, impaired memory, loss of sensation and distorted body awareness are overlooked and these features may be mistaken for depression. The psychological impact of the stroke in terms of the degree of disability and its implications for the patient's future need to be assessed. Those who pride their self-sufficient and independent stance may find it hard to accept even a minor disability, while a dependent personality will often be better able to tolerate such limitations. A stroke can also precipitate an endogenous type depression in those who have a familial history of depression. Treatment involves ensuring that the patient is having adequate rehabilitation therapy for his specific deficit. Patients need to be encouraged to reorganise their lifestyles to allow for the physical disability. A positive therapeutic approach can do much to help and the support and encouragement of the family is essential. Tricyclic antidepressants are frequently useful particularly where there are endogenous features and they will also benefit those with emotional lability associated with pseudobulbar palsy.

Lishman W A 1978 Cerebrovascular disorders. In: Organic Psychiatry. Blackwell, Oxford

229   There are four defined types: delta rhythms at less than 4 cycles per second; theta at 4–7 C/S; alpha rhythms at 8–13 C/S and beta rhythms run in excess of 13 C/S. The normal EEG has a well developed alpha rhythm which is maximal over the posterior half of the scalp and it attenuates when the eyes are open, or when the person is engaged in mental activity. In most subjects the alpha rhythm remains stable. Beta waves are sometimes found in the precentral regions and theta and delta activity will become more obvious with relaxation and drowsiness. Delta activity is normally seen only in very young children and during sleep. The EEG pattern and activity is generally stable for an individual between the ages of 20 and 60 years. Prior to that slow waves predominate and there is great variation both within and between subjects. In infants the waves

are of low voltage and there are irregular and asynchronous theta and delta components. At 18 months the alpha rhythm begins to appear and between 2 and 12 years the recording is polyrhythmic with equal amounts of theta and alpha activity being present at 5 years of age. After 60 years there is often a slowing of the alpha rhythm or a reduction in its amplitude and slow waves frequently appear with advancing years.

Kiloh L G, McComas A J, Osselton J W 1979, Normal findings. In: Clinical Electroencephalography 3rd edn. Butterworth, London

McClelland R 1979 Psychiatric manifestations of organic illness. In: Hill P, Murray R, Thorley A (eds) Essentials of Postgraduate Psychiatry, 1st edn. Academic Press, London

Mullen P E 1986 The mental state and states of mind. In: Hill P, Murray R, Thorley A (eds) Essentials of Postgraduate Psychiatry 2nd edn. Grune and Stratton, London

230   Most phenothiazines have a marked antiadrenergic activity. Thioridazine in particular with its piperidine side chain and chlorpromazine can produce severe postural hypotension with compensatory tachycardia to which tolerance may develop. Orthostatic hypotension may be particularly marked in the elderly. Phenothiazines also have an antiarrhythmic effect on the heart, displaying a quinidine-like action which may antagonise the effects of digoxin. A variety of electrocardiographic changes may be seen, especially with thioridazine, which produces alterations in the configuration of the T-wave. The strongly muscarinic nature of thioridazine may lead to the development of ejaculatory impotence. Anticholinergic manifestations include blurring of vision, dry mouth, constipation and difficulty in micturition.

Hollister L 1984 Drug treatment of schizophrenia. In: Lake C (ed) The Psychiatric Clinics of North America. Clinical Psychopharmacology. September 1984: 435–453.

Saunders, Philadelphia Silverstone T, Turner P 1982 Drug Treatment in Psychiatry, 3rd edn. Routledge & Kegan Paul, London

231   School refusers tend to be timid, inhibited and dependent coming from families with a higher incidence of neurosis. They have less experience

of parental absence in childhood, are of normal or superior intelligence and show exemplary behaviour when at school. Children referred for truancy generally come from larger families and from lower socio-economic groups, are under-achievers educationally and more often have experienced parental absence in infancy and child-hood. The sex incidence is equal in school refusal but boys are more likely to be truants. Emotional upset in truancy is usually conspicuous by its absence and in particular there are no difficulties about leaving the mother at home or venturing into strange situations. Truancy is usually one symptom of a conduct disorder whereas depression, phobias and separation anxiety frequently underlie school refusal. Youngsters who truant often go to elaborate pretences to keep their parents from finding out that they are away from school, while in school refusal the parents are aware of the child's absence from school. Children who refuse to attend school often withdraw from their peer group and become more isolated whereas truancy may involve one child who goes off alone or with others.

Hersov L A 1960(a) Persistent non-attendance at school. Journal of Child Psychology Psychiatry 1: 130–136
Hersov L A 1960(b) Refusal to go to school. Journal of Child Psychology Psychiatry 1: 137–145
Hersov L 1985 School refusal. In: Rutter M, Hersov L (eds) Child and Adolescent Psychiatry, 2nd edn. Blackwell, Oxford

232 The history is of an insidious onset of memory loss with early loss of insight and a steadily progressive course. There is usually a history of forgetting names and faces and a tendency to lose familiar possessions. Errors of judgement at work and inappropriate behaviour are seen, interests wane and a decline in practical performance is noted. Frank depressive or paranoid illnesses may present at an early stage. Dysphasic errors are common but may be subtle; apraxia and spatial agnosia render the patient unable to cope with daily tasks such as dressing, finding the way around the house or doing household tasks. The coarse physical signs of hemiparesis and sensory loss are infrequent but more subtle apraxias, agnosias and dysphasia are seldom missing. Characteristic focal signs include dysgraphia, visual and spatial agnosia, apraxia of face, tongue

and hands, hypokinesis and other Parkinsonian signs. Grand mal seizures are common in the later stages. There is progressive impairment in speech and writing with a concurrent progressive memory loss. Emotional lability is frequently observed with patients demonstrating a 'catastrophic reaction' when taxed beyond their ability. The end stage is one of profound loss of all faculties, total memory loss, incontinence, emaciation and gross neurological deficits.

Lishman W A 1978 Senile dementia, presenile dementia and pseudodementia. In: Organic Psychiatry. Blackwell, Oxford

233 The prevalence of severe dementias is in the range of 3 to 5% in those aged sixty-five and over. In addition the Newcastle study showed that a further 5% had mild mental deterioration. Surveys show increasing prevalence of dementias with advancing age, with rates for severe dementia being less than 3% in the age group sixty- five to sixty-nine, increasing to 20% and above in the eighty-five and over age groups. Most studies show a greater prevalence for women though the arteriosclerotic brain syndromes are found to be more common in men. The prevalence of dementias is significantly higher among the hospitalised elderly than the general population, with rates varying from 12 to 65% in psychiatric hospitals and nursing homes. However, the majority of demented elderly people are resident in the community.

Kay D, Beamish P, Roth M 1964(a) Old age mental disorders in Newcastle-upon-Tyne, Part I. A study of prevalence. British Journal of Psychiatry 110: 146–158
Kay D, Bergmann K 1980 Epidemiology of mental disorders among the aged in the community. In: Birren J, Sloane R (eds) Handbook of Mental Health and Aging. Prentice-Hall, New Jersey

234 As this tends to occur in most instances within 48 hours of cessation or reduction in alcohol consumption and is considered to be a withdrawal state, the usual routine of sedation with chlordiazepoxide, ensuring adequate hydration, giving vitamin supplements and nursing in a quiet environment are the main aspects of treatment. Phenothiazine medication will also be necessary. The nature of the condition means that the patient

will probably need admission to hospital. In over 90% of instances the hallucinations are short lived and usually the phenothiazines can be phased out after 7 to 14 days. Those who go on to have chronic hallucinations will need maintenance phenothiazine medication as their illness is akin to that of schizophrenia.

Hore B D 1976 Psychiatric morbidity. In: Alcohol Dependence. Butterworth, London

235 The main indication of social skills training is for individuals who have difficulties forming and maintaining relationships, who are inhibited, indecisive, lacking in self-confidence and unable to plan effectively. Some degree of training can be used in the majority of psychiatric patients. The training can be a useful part of a rehabilitation programme for long term psychiatric and mentally handicapped patients. It is most useful for those who have incapacitating interpersonal difficulties, neurosis, depression, alcoholism or sexual deviations. Techniques may also be used in hostile, aggressive people in an effort to teach them more appropriate behaviour.

Cobb J 1986 Behavioural psychotherapy. In: Hill P, Murray R, Thorley A (eds) Essentials of Postgraduate Psychiatry 2nd Edn. Grune and Stratton, London

236 In some 90% of such instances the EEG tracing is abnormal. The recording usually shows bilateral slow wave activity of lower amplitude than that seen with abscesses or brain tumours and the pattern of activity may vary from day to day, depending on the alterations in level of consciousness. In the majority of instances the location of the haematoma can be identified from the tracing. Typically there is diminished amplitude or suppression of alpha rhythms with some irregular slow wave activity over the affected side. In some cases there is an attenuation over all of the ipsilateral hemisphere and the contralateral side may then appear more normal.

Kiloh L G, McComas A J, Osselton J W 1979 Space occupying lesions. In: Clinical Electroencephalography. Butterworth, London
McClelland R 1979 Psychiatric manifestations of organic illness. In: Hill P, Murray R, Thorley A (eds) Essentials of Postgraduate Psychiatry 1st edn. Academic Press, London

237 Organic brain reactions are the most common cerebral manifestations of SLE and they occur in some 30% of patients. They are usually acute episodes lasting hours to days and often coincide with systemic relapses. The features are: varying degrees of memory disturbance, to full blown delirium with delusion and auditory and visual hallucinations. These states are often misdiagnosed as schizophrenia when the confusion is not obvious. On rare occasions a chronic dementing picture is evident. Less commonly psychotic depressive, schizophrenic and occasionally manic states are seen, but there is often some minor organic feature present. Some 10% have severe chronic depressions. A depersonalisation syndrome has also been mentioned in connection with SLE. Anxiety and depressive reactions seem to be particularly common and are not solely related to either systemic disability or cortical infarct or haemorrhage. It is now known that antibrain antibodies and a breakdown of the blood-brain barrier leads to the development of an autoimmune encephalitis in this disorder and this probably accounts for some of the cerebral manifestations.

Cutting J, McClelland R 1986 The psychiatric manifestations of organic illness. In: Hill P, Murray R, Thorley A (eds) Essentials of Postgraduate Psychiatry 2nd edn. Grune and Stratton, London
Guez S B 1967 The occurrence of psychiatric illness in systemic lupus erythematosis. American Journal of Psychiatry 123: 1562–1570

238 Because of the many and varied presentations of grief reactions, no one treatment is appropriate and effective in every case. Where alcohol dependence, depressive and phobic disorders or schizophreniform symptoms develop following a bereavement they should be treated by standard methods. Antidepressant medication should only be used for major depressive symptoms which persist unduly and brief hospitalisation may be indicated for the suicidal depressed patient. The prescribing of tranquillisers and hypnotics should be judicious and on a short term basis. Much emphasis has been placed on the importance of bringing about the expression of grief as a means of facilitating the work of mourning. 'Linking objects', for example personal possessions of the dead person, have been used as a means of

provoking mourning. Other methods of dealing with grief include, the inhibition of painful thoughts by actively avoiding reminders of the deceased, selective forgetting and idealisation. Liebermann described a procedure called 'forced mourning' in which the patient is encouraged to express strong feelings as the therapist explores the relationship with the deceased. Personal possessions of the deceased are brought to the sessions and discussed. In the final stage the patient reviews the relationship, stops any avoidance behaviour and adjusts to a new life. It may be important to give permission to the bereaved to stop mourning. Individual, family and group psychotherapy may be used and voluntary support groups may be valuable aids.

Liebermann S 1978 Nineteen cases of morbid grief. British Journal of Psychiatry 132: 159–163
Parkes C M 1985 Bereavement. British Journal of Psychiatry 146: 11–18

239 It has been the most popular of the projective tests and it consists of ten symmetrical inkblots printed on separate cards, five of which are coloured and the rest being achromatic. In analysing and interpreting responses to the cards major emphasis is placed on the way the subject responds, in addition to the content of the responses. For example, a response that reverses the figure—ground relationship or concentrates on a minute section of the blot would be judged differently from conventional responses. No one manner of responding is by itself considered better than others and it is the total pattern of responses that are considered significant. In addition to the size and location of the blot segments responded to, the form, colour, shading and texture noted by the subject and whether movement is perceived is assessed. Research into the validity and reliability of these aspects of the test have been scanty and those investigations that have been carried out cast doubt on its reliability as a measuring instrument. While the initial use of the Rorschach was to analyse personality structure, some believe that it is also an aid in psychiatric diagnosis. In this respect it is thought to be helpful in detecting incipient psychosis that may not be clinically obvious. In recent years the Rorschach has been used less and this seems related to its subjective

nature and the absence of supporting validity and reliability data.

Garfield S L 1975 Personality appraisal. In: Clinical Psychology. Edward Arnold, London

240 Presuming that unilateral treatment is as effective as the bilateral form the indication for its use is the same: severe or resistant depression with endogenous features, chemotherapy resistant manic states and schizoaffective disorders. Unilateral ECT is particularly helpful in elderly depressed patients and in those who complain of memory disturbance following bilateral treatment. While there is a general consensus that unilateral treatment to the non-dominant hemisphere produces less memory disturbance and is associated with more rapid post-ictal recovery, many clinicians believe that the advantages gained are outweighed by the superior antidepressant effect of the bilateral form. D'Elia and Raotma (1975), reviewing studies in this area, reported that in two studies unilateral treatment was more effective, in 14 studies they were found to be equally effective and in 12 bilateral ECT were superior. The most usual placement of the unilateral electrodes is on the non-dominant hemisphere, with the lower electrode being placed 4 cms. above the mid-point of a line joining the lateral angle of the orbit to the external auditory meatus and the upper electrode is applied 9 cms. higher and posteriorly, with the line joining the electrodes making a 70° angle with the line joining the external auditory meatus and the lateral angle of the eye.

D'Elia G, Raotma H 1975 Is unilateral ECT less effective than bilateral ECT? British Journal of Psychiatry 126: 83–89
Fraser M 1982 Memory and electrode placement. In: ECT, a clinical guide. Wiley, Chichester

241 The general aims are to restore normal body weight and eating patterns and to facilitate emotional maturation. The main phases of a treatment programme consist of establishing a trusting relationship with the patient, restoring body weight and then using techniques to promote maturation and personal change within the patient. Weight restoration may simply require advice, support and encouragement. Some patients require hospitalisation where management generally involves a structured ward

environment, skilled nursing care, a high calorie diet and a behavioural approach whereby rewards are earned by weight gain. Drugs such as phenothiazines, tricyclic antidepressants, lithium, appetite stimulants such as cyproheptadine, metoclopramide and L-dopa have been used but their usefulness has not yet been established. Calorie intake varies from two thousand to five thousand calories in different programmes. Bed rest is usually part of the programme with increasing amounts of exercise allowed as weight is gradually restored. The third phase involves psychotherapeutic and educative procedures. Information about the disorder is given to the patient and the family. Psychotherapeutic approaches may be supportive or interpretive and group, individual and family therapeutic interventions can be useful when tailored. Family assessment and family meals play a central role in some programmes. Cognitive behavioural approaches have been used especially in the management of binging and vomiting. Menstruation usually recommences with restoration of body weight and this may be facilitated with clomiphene.

Fairburn C 1988 Eating disorders. In: Kendell R E, Zealley A K (eds) Companion to Psychiatric Studies, 4th edn. Churchill Livingstone, Edinburgh

Hill P 1986 The psychiatry of adolescence. In: Hill P, Murray R, Thorley A (eds) Essentials of Postgraduate Psychiatry 2nd edn. Grune and Stratton, London

242 The main methods of treatment involve exposure in fantasy and in vivo, modelling, response prevention, thought stopping and thought satiation. Response prevention involves exposing the patient to a contaminated object and preventing him from carrying out the rituals. The patients are encouraged to resist their rituals for several hours at a time. Response prevention is carried out in the presence of stimuli which normally provoke the rituals—for example, dirty hands increase washing rituals. Therapists may use modelling techniques in conjunction with response prevention. Initially sessions are supervised by the therapist but family members may be involved as co-therapists. Eventually response prevention is self-imposed. Studies have shown that up to 75% of patients will improve with this treatment and follow-up surveys show that gains are maintained for at least three years. Thought stopping and

thought satiation are the two main behavioural techniques used for obsessional ruminations. In thought stopping, the patient learns to interrupt a train of obsessional thoughts with a sudden distracting stimulus. This may be induced by means of an elastic band worn around the wrist to interrupt the ruminations. Thought satiation, a form of exposure in fantasy, involves encouraging the patient to verbalise his ruminations until the patient is tired. The results are still uncertain. Systematic desensitisation, relaxation therapies, covert sensitisation and paradoxical intention have all been used in treating obsessional disorders.

Marks I M 1981 Cure and care of neuroses. Theory and practice of behavioural psychotherapy. Wiley, New York

Thorley A 1986 Neuroses and personality disorder. In: Hill P, Murray R, Thorley A (eds) Essentials of Postgraduate Psychiatry 2nd edn. Grune and Stratton, London

243 These drugs may cause dry mouth, blurring of vision, sweating, precipitate urinary retention, especially in the elderly with prostatic hypertrophy and exacerbate glaucoma. They decrease the anti-psychotic effect of the phenothiazines, perhaps by decreasing plasma levels. The latter is thought to result from its effect on gut motility and enhancement of phenothiazine metabolism. A major concern is that they may uncover or exacerbate tardive dyskinesia and a direct role in causation of this syndrome has been postulated. The drugs themselves may produce a choreiform dyskinesia. Euphoric effects of these drugs may lead to dependency and abuse. They may in susceptible people cause an organic psychosis characterised by delirium, hallucinations and restlessness. An atropinic psychosis may be precipitated by interaction of the anticholinergic drugs and some phenothiazines with strong atropinic properties. Psychometric impairment has been demonstrated in non-psychiatric, non-demented geriatric patients taking small doses of anticholinergics.

McClelland H 1986 Treatment in schizophrenia: Overview. In: Kerr A, Snaith P (eds) Contemporary Issues in Schizophrenia. Gaskell Psychiatry Series

Silverstone T, Turner P 1982 Drug treatment in psychiatry 3rd edn. Routledge & Kegan Paul, London

244 It is important not to assume that the diagnosis is conversion hysteria in view of the fact that an underlying organic explanation for the symptom may later become apparent. A detailed history should be taken from the patient and a relative to establish the time of onset of the symptoms, its nature and constancy, presence of recent stressful life events and whether there is an element of secondary gain from the complaint. This should be followed by a comprehensive physical examination. If the symptoms and signs correspond to the patients idea of what they should be, rather than what they can be in pathophysiological terms, if there is no positive evidence to support an organic explanation and if the symptoms can be explained in terms of a psychological conflict then a diagnosis of hysteria can be made. The patient and relatives should receive a simple explanation of the emotional conflict and how it produced the symptom. This will allay their anxiety, lessening the tendency for the conversion process to be self perpetuating. Against this background certain medical investigations can be performed without reinforcing the patient's impression of it being a medical disorder. Further management will usually involve exploring the emotional conflict through psychotherapy. An interview conducted with intravenous sodium amytal or under hypnosis may provide a rapid access to the particular psychodynamics.

Thorley A 1986 Neurosis and personality disorder. In: Hill P, Murray R, Thorley A (eds) Essentials of Postgraduate Psychiatry 2nd edn. Grune and Stratton, London

245 The outcome is generally poor in terms of intellectual development, overall adjustment and work potential. In adult life, some two-thirds of autistic individuals are still severely handicapped and are unable to look after themselves with the majority residing in long stay institutions. Approximately 5 to 15% are working and have gained some measure of a social life. Even those who do become independent show continuing difficulties in relationships and oddities of personality. The prognosis is strongly associated with the IQ and the degree of language development. The 30% of individuals who have an IQ above 70 comprise the majority of those who improve most. Convulsions occur for the first time in up to 30% during

adolescence and the risk is considerably higher for those with severe mental retardation. Approximately one half of autistic individuals gain useful speech and a better outcome is associated with the development of functional speech before the age of five. The child becomes more responsive with increasing speech development. Even in those who achieve near normal language competence a peculiar pedantic style exists with residual difficulties with rhythm and abstract concepts. Mutism indicates a poor prognosis. While about 50% show improvement in their sociability, relationships usually remain abnormal and they generally remain reserved, aloof, lack interpersonal skills and have difficulty in empathising and maintaining relationships. A small number regress during adolescence, lose language skills and become apathetic.

Kolvin I 1982 Outcome and prognosis of early childhood psychoses. In: Wing J, Wing L (eds) Handbook of Psychiatry 3. Psychoses of uncertain aetiology. Cambridge University Press, Cambridge

246 Because of the increased sensitivity of the elderly to the effects of drugs and because of their increased probability of being on more than one drug due to multiple pathology, drug prescribing should be kept to a minimum. One should commence treatment at a low dose, increase slowly, review regularly and arrange for supervision of drug taking. Compliance is a real problem often due to forgetfulness, so less frequent dosage regimens should be the aim. Single daily doses at night time should be feasible but may be hazardous because of cardiotoxic effects following the absorption of a single large dose. Sustained release preparations frequently avoid toxicity. Side effects are generally more pronounced in the elderly. Impairment of renal or liver metabolism result in more potent or prolonged effects and may increase the likelihood of side effects. None of the major tranquillisers are free from dystonic and extrapyramidal side effects and this seriously curtails their use. Anti-Parkinsonian medications produce sedation and this poses a problem in drug administration. Concomitant medication to the elderly who tend to have multiple physical problems must be carefully monitored. Confusion may occur due to over-medication or unsuspected drug interactions. Two or more drugs may interact

additively, synergistically or antagonistically at the same or different receptor sites. Over the counter medication should be kept to a minimum.

Cayley A 1985 Drug prescribing in the elderly. British Journal of Hospital Medicine 34(6): 355–358
Lader M 1982 Psychopharmacology of old age. In: Levy R, Post F (eds) The Psychiatry of Late Life. Blackwell, Oxford

247   The socio-cultural theory proposes that the current emphasis on thinness and the dietary behaviour of adolescents are important aetiological factors. Support for this theory is found in the increasing incidence of anorexia nervosa and the increased prevalence found among dance and modelling students. Psychoanalytic theories see anorexia nervosa as a struggle for self-respecting identity. Bruch stressed the importance of the body image disturbance, the defects in the accuracy of perception of body sensations and the inability to function autonomously. She also described in patients a 'paralysing sense of ineffectiveness' which she attributes to the parents' failure to promote self-expression. Crisp sees the condition as a psychological regression in the face of adolescent conflict. He proposes that the avoidance of food and resulting weight loss lead to abnormalities in the regulation of menstruation and hence regression to a pre-pubertal level of functioning. This theory is supported by the finding of pre-pubertal levels of gonadotrophins and gonadal steroids in anorexic patients. Minuchin maintains that certain types of abnormal family relationships are of importance in the development of anorexia nervosa. He suggests that the individual who is physiologically vulnerable can, in the context of abnormal patterns of family relationships, develop anorexia nervosa and this serves to prevent dissension within the family. There is some evidence to support a genetic aetiology but most twin studies are not large enough to give reliable estimates of concordance. A primary disorder of hypothalamic function could be deduced from the almost invariable feature of amenorrhoea, especially when it precedes weight loss and the other endocrine changes which reflect involvement of the hypothalamic–pituitary–gonadal axis. Turner's syndrome, urogenital abnormalities and perinatal injury all appear to

increase the likelihood of developing anorexia nervosa.

Fairburn C 1988 Eating disorders. In: Kendell R E, Zealley A K (eds) Companion to Psychiatric Studies, 4th edn. Churchill Livingstone, Edinburgh

248 The first step is to discuss the treatment with the patient and acquaint him and his family with the procedure. The patient's written consent is then obtained. Fitness for anaesthesia is then assessed. This involves taking a full medical history and doing a physical examination. Particular attention needs to be given to the cardiac and pulmonary status, dental care, previous anaesthetic history, allergies and family history of anaesthetic complications. A simple test of memory and orientation should be made as a baseline recording. Finally the patient should be instructed not to eat or drink from the midnight of the night before the treatment and for patients who might have difficulty following these instructions because of their mental state their fast needs to be supervised.

Fraser M 1982 Administration of E.C.T. In: ECT, a clinical guide. Wiley, Chichester

249 Pituitary gonadotrophins tend to be present in lower than usual quantities in the circulation of anorexic patients, although follicular stimulating hormone (FSH) is less consistently depressed than luteinizing hormone (LH). The pattern of secretion over 24-hours is also different in anorexic subjects, in that they resemble those of prepubertal girls rather than age matched controls. Anorexic subjects show a markedly diminished or absent LH response to LH releasing hormone and they have either uniformly low or higher plasma LH levels. These patterns are reversed when weight is restored during sleep. The FSH response to releasing hormone is less diminished and is more readily restored by weight gain. Clomiphene, a drug which blocks the negative feedback of oestrogens at the hypothalamic levels, is effective in promoting ovulation and menstruation only when weight has been restored to near normal levels. With weight gain the endocrine abnormalities revert to normal and menstruation returns in all but 10% to 15% of cases, though there is great variation in the

timing. Thyroxine and thyroid stimulating hormone are generally within normal limits though tri-iodothyronine (T3) may be low. There is usually an increase in the inactivated reverse form of T3 but levels return to normal with weight gain. Growth hormone levels are variable although elevated concentrations are seen in acute starvation. Plasma cortisol levels are generally elevated, the diurnal variation in secretion rates is often disturbed and the dexamethasone suppression test is abnormal at low weights. Some subjects show a partial diabetes insipidus probably related to disorder of the posterior pituitary function.

Casper R 1984 Hypothalamic dysfunction and symptoms of anorexia nervosa. In: Larocca F (ed) The Psychiatric Clinics of North America Eating disorders, June 1984: 201–215. Saunders, Philadelphia

Palmer R 1982 Anorexia nervosa. In: Granville–Grossman K (ed) Recent Advances in Clinical Psychiatry 4. Churchill Livingstone, Edinburgh

250 It is a rare disorder in which the patient believes that a person, usually a close relative, has been replaced by an exact double. It is also known as the 'illusion of doubles' (l'illusion des sosils), but more accurately as the 'delusion of doubles'. It is questionable whether it should be regarded as a clear cut syndrome or merely a symptom occurring as part of a recognised psychosis. Though it can occur in isolation, the Capgras delusions usually accompany a paranoid psychosis of either the schizophrenic or affective type and can occur at any stage of these disorders. While cases have been reported where organic factors have been implicated, a comprehensive neuropsychiatric review of 11 patients with the syndrome found that 6 had schizophrenia, 4 had a depressive illness and the remaining patient had a cerebral organic disorder with marked paranoid features. With this delusional syndrome the patient is intellectually aware that there is no difference between the person and the imposter, but projects negative feelings onto the imposter while maintaining positive feelings for the 'absent and real' person. Management involves treating the primary disorder, helping the implicated relative understand the nature of the complaint and endeav-

ouring to resolve the interpersonal conflict between patient and relative.

Enoch D M, Trethowan W H 1979 The Capgras syndrome. In: Uncommon Psychiatric Syndromes. Wright, Bristol

251 Infantile autism, or early childhood psychosis, presents with characteristic abnormalities of social interaction and language. They have typical repetitive and stereotyped behaviour and the disorder has its onset before thirty months. Schizophrenia, by contrast, is very rare before seven years and presents with thought disorder, auditory hallucinations, delusions, blunted affect and perplexity. There is an excess of schizophrenia among the parents of schizophrenic children, while in autism there is no increase in psychopathology among the parents, but 15% of the siblings have language delay. Follow up studies similarly differentiate the two conditions; infantile autism does not develop into schizophrenia, both remaining quite distinct. Organic cerebral dysfunction in autism is well described; one in four autistic adolescents have epilepsy and there is a marked increase in the prevalence of autism among those children with such brain damaged conditions as rubella embryopathy and infantile spasms. Finally, the mean IQ of those with late onset psychosis is within the normal range, while for those with autism approximately 70% have an IQ of less than 70.

Kolvin I 1971 Psychoses in childhood—a comparative study. In: Rutter M (ed) Infantile Autism: Concepts, Characteristics and Treatment 7–26. Churchill Livingstone, Edinburgh
Kolvin I 1982 Outcome and prognosis of early childhood psychoses. In: Wing L, Wing J K (eds) Handbook of Psychiatry 3. Psychoses of uncertain aetiology. Cambridge University Press, Cambridge

252 Psychogeriatric patients are more likely to have low vitamin B12 levels than matched non-psychiatric controls. However, it is uncertain in how many cases the deficiency is the cause rather than the consequence of the cognitive deficit. Surveys of general psychiatric patients tend to indicate that they are likely to have low levels of B12, but the matter is not conclusive as other studies contradict these findings. Minor affective disturbances are common in those with the deficiency and they

may often be the earliest manifestations. However, the causal connection between B12 deficiency and depression has not been firmly established. It is thought that the mood disturbance may be no more than a reaction to the physical illness and that in some instances it may represent a depression which has been precipitated by the deficiency. This fact is emphasised in that the depression often responds before vitamin replacement treatment has started. The aetiological connection between B12 deficiency and cerebral organic reactions is more convincing; in one prospective study some 75% of patients with pernicious anaemia had memory impairment and in the majority of cases the cognitive impairment improved with replacement therapy.

Shulman R 1967 Psychiatric aspects of pernicious anaemia: A prospective controlled investigation. British Medical Journal iii: 266–270

Shulman R 1967 Vitamin B12 deficiency and psychiatric illness. British Journal of Psychiatry 113: 252–256

253 Present day classifications accord more priority to depressive than to anxiety features in that if both are present in equal proportions a depressive illness tends to be diagnosed. Furthermore, anxiety features are only deduced as belonging to a primary anxiety state after depression, phobic disorders, schizophrenia and all other disorder with which anxiety is associated, have been excluded. Anxiety symptoms developing for the first time after the age of 40 tend to indicate the presence of an underlying affective disorder or an extracerebral organic cause. An anxiety state usually presents as an extension of an anxious premorbid personality which has been under stress. If anxiety features appear without any obvious precipitating life event or in a stable personality then the diagnosis is likely to be depression. Roth and his colleagues have concluded from their extensive work on the validation of anxiety and depressive categories that early morning wakening, self-denigration, psychomotor retardation, hopelessness, suicidal tendencies and a remitting pattern indicate a depressive disorder while somatic tension, panic attacks, compulsions, vasomotor instability, derealisation, paranoid and hypochondriacal ideas and histrionic and aggressive behaviour are the

constellation of features associated with anxiety states.

Roth M, Gurney C, Garside R F, Kerr T A 1972
Studies in the classification of affective disorders.
The relationship between anxiety states and
depressive illness. British Journal of Psychiatry
121: 147–161

254 Solvent abuse is mainly a group activity associated with adolescent males. In the USA a life time prevalence of 16.5% for individuals aged 12–17 has been reported and the rates drop to 10% for those aged 18–25 and to 4% for those over 25 years. The prevalence in Britain is still uncertain but a point prevalence of 10% for boys aged 13–15 was found in one survey. Abuse is at least twice as common among boys than girls and their background tends to be one of poor academic achievement, deprived families living in inner city areas and members of rebellious antisocial groups. Outbreaks of abuse have been noted among ethnic minority groups and in specific schools. Peer influence emerges as a major factor and in about two-third of all cases, solvent abuse is a group activity. Solitary adolescents who sniff glue do so to become intoxicated and euphoric and they are more likely to become dependent and develop serious side effects. They have backgrounds with greater levels of family disruptions, parental absence and alcoholism.

Herzeberg J, Wolkind S 1983 Solvent sniffing in
perspective. British Journal Hospital Medicine
29: 72–76
Ramsey A W 1982 Solvent abuse: An educational
perspective. Human Toxicology 1: 265–270
Watson J M 1980 Solvent abuse by children and
young adults. British Journal of Addition 75: 27–36

255 Negativism is an apparently motiveless resistance to suggestion or attempts at movement. Fish has described an active and passive form. In the active form the patient does the exact opposite to what is requested or required, while in the passive form all interference is vigorously resisted and any attempt to force the patient to do something is met with increasing resistance. Severe excitement may occur if attempts are made to force the patient to do something or to prevent him from carrying out a spontaneous act. Negativism occurs in catatonic schizophrenia, in severe mental handi-

cap and in dementia. The resistance to suggestion that is encountered in other psychiatric disorders is understandable in the context of the person's thought content and is not a form of negativism.

Hamilton M (ed) 1984 Fish's clinical psychopathology, 3rd edn. Wright, Bristol

256 The optimal rate of reduction of benzodiazepines is uncertain, though abrupt withdrawal is more likely to lead to serious symptoms, including epileptic seizures. In most uncomplicated cases, gradual withdrawal on an out-patient basis will suffice. As the severity of the withdrawal reaction is probably more closely related to the rate of reduction of the drug levels rather than the absolute levels, it may be advisable to change from a short acting to a long acting benzodiazepine as this will result in a more gradual fall. Beta blocking drugs may reduce the severity of the symptoms and the adrenergic blocking effect of clonidine may be helpful. Sedative tricyclic drugs such as amitriptyline or other drugs such as chlormetiazole may have a role but their use should be carefully supervised. Many psychological treatments have been advocated and they include supportive psychotherapy, cognitive therapy, relaxation and anxiety management techniques. Group therapy is currently in vogue but the results are disappointing.

Petursson H, Lader M H 1981 Withdrawal from long term benzodiazepine treatment. British Medical Journal 283: 643–645
Tyrer P 1984 Benzodiazepines on trial. British Medical Journal 288 (6424): 1101–1102

257 No. While clearly there is a place for short-term prescription, these drugs should only be used for significant extrapyramidal side effects. The prevalence of these side effects range from 23% to 88% of patients taking neuroleptics, but most studies cluster around a 40% rate. Many studies have found these drugs to be unnecessary and ineffective in a substantial proportion of patients. Because many patients seem to develop tolerance to the neurological side effects, many authorities suggest that anticholinergics should be used only for the duration of the side effects. Surveys indicate that only a minority develop neurological symptoms after discontinuation of the anticholinergics. Up to two-thirds of the extrapyramidal

symptoms can be abolished by dose reduction of the phenothiazine alone. Anticholinergic agents may also precipitate an organic psychosis which is exacerbated by the atropinic properties of the phenothiazines. They also reduce the plasma levels of phenothiazines through enzyme induction and changes in gut motility. Anticholinergic agents in themselves may produce a choreiform dyskinesia and may uncover or exacerbate tardive dyskinesia.

Hollister L 1984 Drug treatment of schizophrenia. In: Lake C (ed) The Psychiatric Clinics of North America Clinical Psychopharmocology. September 1984. 435–453. Saunders, Philadelphia

McClelland A 1986 Treatment of schizophrenia: Overview. In: Kerr A, Snaith P (eds) Contemporary Issues in Schizophrenia. Gaskell Psychiatry Series

258   Tramer coined the term to describe a group of children who speak only with a small group of intimates in very specific situations, such as in the home. It is a rare disorder with a prevelance of 0.8 per 1,000 and it has a female predominance. Commonly mutism comes to attention when the child starts school, the usual pattern being that the child speaks at home but not at school. While it is considered a motivational disorder, recent research shows evidence of articulation defects, EEG immaturities, speech delay and sphincter difficulties. These children also exhibit low non-verbal intelligence, poor peer relationships, separation difficulties, a range of behavioural problems and adverse temperamental traits. There is evidence of an early insidious onset of shyness and approximately 50% show a pattern of sulky, aggressive behaviour. Their parents frequently have psychiatric disorders and deviant personalities. Follow-up studies reveal that approximately half improve in both speech and social adjustment, irrespective of the treatment they receive.

Kolvin I, Fundudis T 1981 Elective mute children: Psychological development and background factors. Journal of Child Psychology and Psychiatry 22: 219–232

Kolvin I, Goodyear I 1982 Child psychiatry. In: Granville–Grossman K (ed) Recent Advances in Clinical Psychiatry 4. Churchill Livingstone, Edinburgh

259   Many drugs have been used in the prevention and alleviation of dementia but when carefully tested,

most have proved disappointing. Vasodilators are the main group of drugs that have been applied. In multi-infarct dementia they do not reverse atherosclerotic changes nor improve perfusion through occluded vessels. Theoretically they can act on anastomotic communications round the periphery of infarcts but there is a real risk of a 'steal' effect which could worsen the clinical picture. They are of two types: primary vasodilators and those with vasodilator and metabolic actions. Cyclandelate, a primary vasodilator often causes side effects of nausea, flushing and rashes and its value has not been demonstrated. Codergocrine mesylate has been claimed by many to show improvement on behavioural and psychological tests but clinically it has not been shown to be of much benefit. Dihydroergotoxine is widely used but any improvements noted have not been substantial. Central nervous stimulants such as methylphenidate are often used but again these drugs do not produce any worthwhile improvement in cognitive function and have many adverse effects. Because of the demonstrated cholinergic defect in Alzheimer's disease it was hoped that drugs which increase acetylcholine levels might rectify the deficiency. Agents in this category include precursor loading with choline and lecithin, gamma-amino-butyric acid derivatives such as piracetam which accelerates acetylcholine release and physostigmine a cholinesterase inhibitor. However, while short term improvement has been reported the value of these preparations is still unproven. Peptides such as vasopressin, desmopressin and procaine have also been tried.

Gurland B, Birkett D 1983 The senile and presenile dementias. In: Lader M (ed) Handbook of Psychiatry 2. Mental disorders and somatic illness. Cambridge University Press, Cambridge

260 Hobson (1953), in a study of uncategorised depressives found that a good response was associated with an onset of depression within eight weeks of the treatment, good insight, obsessional personality, self-reproach and psychomotor retardation. Carney and his colleagues (1965) found that weight loss, pyknic build, early morning wakening, somatic and paranoid delusions were favourable indices and they were able to predict the correct therapeutic response in 87% of cases. Evening worsening of symptoms, hypochondriacal, anxiety and hysterical features and self pity

predicted a poor therapeutic outcome. A more recent study at Northwick Park found that only delusions predicted a favourable response and that retardation and other favourable predictive features noted in previous studies were not useful. However, the small sample size and the type of patient studied might account for this negative finding.

Carney M W P, Roth M, Garside R F 1965 The diagnosis of depressive syndromes and the prediction of ECT response. British Journal of Psychiatry 111: 659–674

Hobson R F 1953 Prognostic factors in electroconvulsive therapy. Journal of Neurology, Neurosurgery and Psychiatry 16: 275–281

Northwick Park ECT Trial 1984 Predictors of response to real and simulated ECT. British Journal of Psychiatry 144: 227–237

261 This is a technique in which the individual, by being made aware of changes in his physiological functions by means of electronic instruments, can learn to regulate these changes voluntarily. It involves the conversion of physiological data, such as heart rate, blood pressure, EEG activity, muscle tension and skin temperature, into visual or audible signals. Its use has been explored with tension headaches, chronic pain, migraine, hypertension and anxiety states. EEG feedback may be useful in treating insomnia and some forms of epilepsy. Electromyographic feedback may be used to treat faecal incontinence and neuromuscular disorders. Other indications include tics and spasms. Bell's palsy, peripheral nerve damage and training blind people to adopt appropriate facial expressions. Although it can be shown to be more effective than control procedures, it has not been established that it is superior to simpler behavioural techniques such as relaxation therapy.

Kogeorgos J, Scott D 1981 Biofeedback and its clinical applications. British Journal Hospital Medicine June 25: 601–605

Yates A J 1980 Biofeedback and the modification of behaviour. Plenum, New York

262 Research into prevalence and incidence rates is hampered by the tendency of these patients to deny their symptoms and because of the uncertainty over how to designate mild cases. Case register studies yield an annual incidence rate ranging from 0.24 to 1.6 per 100,000 population

and suggest that there is an increasing incidence of the illness over the past few decades. Theander in Sweden found an overall incidence of 0.24 per 100,000 population for a thirty year period. However, the rate for the third decade (1951–1960) was higher at 0.45 cases per 100,000 population. Kendall reporting on the findings of three psychiatric registers showed an incidence rate varying from 0.37 per 100,000 to 1.6 per 100,000. Crisp found a prevalence rate of one in one hundred girls aged sixteen or older who were attending English public schools, but only one in three thousand among girls attending comprehensive schools. Other workers have noted an increase in rates for anorexia nervosa in university students. Garner and Garfinkel found a particularly high prevalence rate among particular groups—6.5% prevalence rate in dance students and 7% among modelling students.

Palmer R 1982 Anorexia nervosa. In: Granville-Grossman K (ed) Recent Advances in Clinical Psychiatry. Churchill Livingstone, Edinburgh

263 Asperger in 1944 described a personality type characterised by impaired social relationships, lack of empathy, constricted and unusual interests and an odd pedantic use of language. The basis for the solitariness is felt to be an inability to make relationships due to a lack of sensitivity and a deficit in normal verbal and non-verbal communication. Boys are predominantly affected and results of follow-up studies into early adulthood indicate that they continue to be distinguishable from normal young adults. There is commonly a history of similar, though less extreme, characteristics in their fathers, an excess of adverse perinatal experiences and sometimes developmental anomalies including language delay. When compared with intelligent autistic children and normal children they appear to fall into an intermediate category.

Wing L 1979 Asperger's syndrome: A clinical account. Psychological Medicine 11: 115–129
Wolff S, Chick J 1980 Schizoid personality in childhood: A controlled follow up study. Psychological Medicine 10: 85–100

264 There are no clear cut indications for psychosurgery but it is mainly used in the management of

intractable depression, chronic anxiety and disabling obsessive compulsive neurosis. There are reports of psychosurgery being used in those with aggressive behaviour, sexual deviancy and psychopathic personalities, but its use is both highly controversial and of questionable value. Although prefrontal leucotomy was originally introduced for the treatment of neurosis some two-thirds of the 10,000 operations of this type performed in Britain between 1942 and 1952 were for schizophrenia. Since the advent of neuroleptics, psychosurgery has been performed infrequently for this disorder and then only where disabling anxiety, depressive or obsessive features persist despite chemotherapy. In general psychosurgery should only be considered when the disabling target symptoms have been shown to be resistant to chemotherapy, ECT and psychotherapy and have been present for a long period. Of what duration and severity the symptoms experienced should be before the patient is considered for psychosurgery is uncertain. From the limited data available in Britain it appears that the majority of subjects operated on have been ill for at least two years and have failed to respond to a wide range of conventional treatments.

Mitchell–Heggs N, Kelly D, Richardson A 1976
Stereotactic limbic leucotomy—a follow up at 16 months. British Journal of Psychiatry 128: 226–240

265 Ganser described a syndrome of which the most prominent feature was the tendency to give approximate answers to simple questions and the word 'Vorbeigehen' or to 'pass by' has been used to describe the phenomenon. Examples of approximate answers would be that the sum of 2 plus 2 equals 5, or that the cat has five legs. Other features of the syndrome are clouding of consciousness, somatic and conversion symptoms and psychogenic hallucinations. The clouding of consciousness is evident by the patient's bewildered appearance and he may be semi-stuporose and disorientated. The memory disturbance tends to be more like a psychogenic amnesia in that it abates when the person is away from the troubled situation. The hallucinations may be auditory or visual and their content pertains to the subject's life situation. While the syndrome is extremely rare, Ganser symptoms, or a tendency to give approximate answers, is frequently seen in connection with functional and organic psychoses.

The Ganser syndrome is generally considered to be a hysterical dissociative state which occurs as a result of an unconscious effort by the subject to escape an intolerable situation.

Cutting J 1986 Atypical psychosis. In: Hill P, Murray R, Thorley A (eds) Essentials of Postgraduate Psychiatry 2nd edn. Grune and Stratton, London
Enoch D M, Trethowan W H 1979 The Ganser syndrome. In: Uncommon Psychiatric Syndromes. Wright, Bristol

266 Stupor is a state of complete psychomotor inhibition with retention of consciousness in which the patient shows profound lack of responsiveness and mutism. Total stupor of this severity is uncommon; milder forms are more often encountered. The patient may lie or sit motionless and will not respond to commands, but from time to time his facial expression may change in response to what is being said or done. In catatonic states the patient may adopt bizarre postures and impulsive actions may also occur. While spontaneous movement is generally not evident, the patient will respond to painful stimuli. Unlike comatose states the patient may stare at the examiner or follow him, or objects, in the room with his eyes. When his eyes are shut they may resist passive opening. Sphincter control is variable; there may be retention or incontinence of both urine and faeces. Neurological signs may be absent, but this will depend on the aetiology of the stuporose state. Causes can be organic or functional in origin. Functional causes include depression, catatonic schizophrenia, mania, hysterical or psychogenic stupor. Organic causes include diencephalon or mid-brain tumours, neurosyphilis, encephalitis lethargica and senile or presenile dementias. Extracranial causes which may occasionally present include renal failure, hypothyroidism, hypopituitarism, hyperparathyroidism and water intoxication. Alcoholic and barbiturate intoxication, hypoglycaemia and dehydration with electrolyte disturbances have also been implicated.

Johnson J 1982 Stupor. Its diagnosis and management. British Journal of Hospital Medicine. May 530–532
Lishman W A 1978 Differential diagnosis. In: Organic Psychiatry. Blackwell, Oxford

267 The principal features are CNS dysfunction, which may be intellectual, behavioural or neuro-

logical, pre- and post-natal growth deficiency, characteristic facial abnormalities and major organ anomalies. The facial manifestations are very variable and the eyes, nose, mouth and mandible are mainly affected. Features which may be present include epicanthal folds, strabismus, severe myopia, cleft palate, short nasal tip and dental malocclusion secondary to a flat mid face and prominent mandible. Cardiac abnormalities such as atrial septal defects, skeletal disorders such as dislocated hips and neurological defects are common features though any organ may be affected. Irritability and moderate mental retardation are the most frequent CNS abnormalities. An incidence of 1 to 2 per 1,000 live births, with partial expression in another 3 to 5 births, has been reported. The risk of development of the syndrome is proportional to the average daily alcohol intake: over 80 g of alcohol daily poses a major threat though there are sufficient grounds to accept that daily intake of 20 to 80 g may be harmful.

Archives of disease in childhood 1984 Editorial. Alcohol and the Foetus 59: 1113–1114

Streissguth A, Clarren S, Jones R 1985 Natural history of the foetal alcohol syndrome: A 10 year follow up of eleven patients. Lancet 85–91 July

268 This is a psychotic state occurring in severe hypothyroidism and the term was coined in 1949 by Richard Asher. It is generally agreed that there is no one specific form of the psychosis and that the clinical picture is one of a variety of different reaction types, which vary from one individual to another. The most common form is an organic psychosis which is usually acute and presents with delusions of persecution, hallucinations, mental confusion and impairment of consciousness. Sometimes the cognitive disturbance runs a subacute or chronic course and presents as dementia. In other instances a schizophrenic or a depressive psychosis is the mode of presentation, but evidence of cerebral organic symptoms will be found if carefully sought. Paranoid delusions which are frequently quite bizarre tend to colour both the organic and functional syndromes.

Asher R 1949 Myxoedematous Madness. British Medical Journal 2: 555–562

Tonks C M 1964 Mental illness in hypothyroid patients. British Journal of Psychiatry 110: 706–710

269 Cortisol hypersecretion occurs during some depressive illnesses and this reflects a hypersecretion of adrenocorticotropic hormone and corticotrophic releasing factor. The dexamethasone suppression test (DST) is used to test the suppressability of cortisol hypersecretion, as dexamethasone normally impairs cortisol output by blocking adrenocorticotropic hormone release. Patients who have a depressive syndrome without disturbance of variables such as sleep, appetite and psychomotor function have normal rates of cortisol secretion and have a negative DST response. Carroll claims that the test has an overall specificity of 96% and a sensitivity of 43%, in other words that the test can be used with a high degree of confidence to support a diagnosis of melancholia or endogenous depression, but a negative test will not necessarily exclude this diagnosis. More recently there have been reports from other investigators which failed to show that it had diagnostic specificity and positive test results have been found in senile dementia, schizophrenia, neurotic states, anorexia nervosa and abstinent alcoholics. Until further data is available the usefulness of the DST in psychiatric practise will remain uncertain.

Carroll B J 1982 The dexamethasone suppression test for melancholia. British Journal of Psychiatry 140: 292–304

Coppen A, Abou–Saleh M, Milln P, Metcalfe M, Harwood J, Bailey J 1983 The dexamethasone suppression test in depression and other psychiatric illness. British Journal of Psychiatry 142: 498–504

270 The most widely used hallucinogen is LSD (lysergic acid diethylamide). Others include hallucinogenic mushrooms, mescaline, DOM (25-dimethoxy-4-methyl amphetamine) phencyclidine and psilocybin. LSD's action is rapid. Its duration of action is variable and it may last up to twelve hours. Tolerance usually develops rapidly and disappears after a few days of abstinence. LSD does not produce physical dependence. Autonomic effects appear early with pupil dilation, increased body temperature, tachycardia and tremor. Other physical symptoms include lacrimation, salivation, paresthesia and a mild leucocytosis. Affective disturbance is varied and extensive, and while euphoria is usually the predominant mood, paranoia, depression, agitation

and panic may follow and constitute a 'bad trip'. Much depends on the subject's premorbid personality, his expectations and the setting in which the drug is being taken. Perceptual distortions, illusions and pseudohallucinations occur mainly in the visual sphere. Auditory perceptions are greatly enhanced. Synaesthesia, the merging of sensory modalities, is often marked and distortion of body image may take bizarre shapes. 'Flashbacks', which are the spontaneous recurrences of LSD effects, may occur during abstinence. A schizophrenic-like psychosis can follow repeated use of the drug but this generally resolves spontaneously on cessation of drug use. Psychotic symptoms are claimed to follow prolonged use but these may be more related to a pre-existing vulnerability rather than a direct drug effect. A toxic effect of LSD on chromosomes has been postulated but it has not been substantiated.

Madden J S 1986 A guide to alcohol and drug dependence. Wright, Bristol

Thorley A 1986 Drug problems. In: Hill P, Murray R, Thorley A (eds) Essentials of Postgraduate Psychiatry 2nd edn. Grune and Stratton, London

271   While brain damaged children do not show any specific psychiatric sequelae, they are more likely to be hyperactive and to have a short attention span. However, the syndrome is compatible with normal intelligence. There is an increased incidence of antisocial personality, hysteria and alcoholism among the first degree relatives of hyperactive children and the biological parents of these children suffer more psychiatric illness than the adoptive parents. Studies of temperament show that the activity level of monozygotic twins is more alike than that of dizygotic twins. These findings all implicate a genetic component. Idiosyncratic reactions to food additives probably have a small role to play in the development of the syndrome. The psychological factors which appear to be relevant are emotional deprivation and maternal depression. Thus a reasonable view of aetiology would have regard for the interaction between genetic factors, family influences and occasionally reactions to environmental toxins.

Taylor E 1985 Syndromes of overactivity and attention deficit. In: Rutter M, Hersov L (eds) Child and Adolescent Psychiatry. Blackwell, Oxford

Weiss G 1985 Hyperactivity: Overview and new
directions. In: Beitchman J (ed) Psychiatric Clinics
of North America. Child Psychiatry, December
1985. Saunders, Philadelphia

272 This is the phenomenon whereby an increased
drug dosage is required to maintain a given drug
effect and it may be innate or acquired. Innate
tolerance is subject to wide individual variation
determined presumably by genetic factors and the
age of the individual. Acquired tolerance may be
of three types: dispositional, pharmacodynamic
and behavioural. Dispositional drug tolerance
refers to pharmacokinetic changes of the drug
within the individual so that there are reduced
drug concentrations at the site of action, often
resulting in increased rates of metabolism. Pharmacodynamic tolerance refers to adaptive changes
within the individual so that the response is
reduced for the same concentration of the drug.
Behavioural tolerance relates to changes in
response due to psychological mechanisms. The
mechanisms underlying the development of tolerance are ill-understood but may include proliferation of new receptor sites or reduction in
sensitivity of receptors to their agonists. Tolerance
does not necessarily occur for all of the effects of
a drug: repeated doses of morphine induces tolerance to the depressant effects of the drug on the
central nervous system but not to its effect on
pupil size or mobility. Tolerance may be, or may
not be, accompanied by physical or psychological
dependence. Cross tolerance may occur among
groups of drugs, such as is seen among the opiates
and the benzodiazepines.

Jaffe J H 1980 Drug addiction and drug abuse. In:
Gilman A G, Goodman L S, Gilman A (eds) The
Pharmacological Basis of Therapeutics 6th edn.
MacMillan, New York
Silverstone T, Turner P 1982 (eds) Drug treatment
in psychiatry, 3rd edn. Routledge & Kegan Paul,
London

273 This is a condition in which the patient does not
speak and makes no attempt at spoken communication, despite preservation of an adequate level
of consciousness. It may be encountered in
disturbed children, organic brain disorders or
functional psychiatric states such as depression,
mania, hysteria and schizophrenia. Catatonic

states are nearly always associated with mutism. Hysterical mutism is very rare. Elective mutism is a motivational disorder seen in children, they speak to intimates only in familiar situations and the mutism usually occurs in school. The term akinetic mutism is a stuporose condition due to a lesion in the central midline structures of the mid-brain and in the diencephalon, such as pinealomas, Rathkes pouch tumours and other space occupying lesions. In akinetic mutism the patients are mute, have an altered level of consciousness and anterograde amnesia. Mutism may be a feature of dementia. Aphasic patients are very rarely mute, as even in the most severe cases of aphasia the patient attempts to communicate using gestures or grunts.

Hamilton M (ed) 1984 Fish's clinical psychopathology, 3rd edn. Wright, Bristol

274 A number of studies have reported that some 30% of depressed patients have a blunted thyroid stimulating hormone (TSH) response to intravenously administered thyrotropin releasing hormone (TRH). The clinical characteristics of those with an impaired TSH response are not clear, but a number of investigations report that unipolar depressives are more likely than bipolar patients to have an impaired response and those who continue to have a blunted response when apparently normothymic are more likely to relapse. Exactly why there is an impaired response is uncertain, but it may be related to increased serum thyroxine levels during depression in some patients or to the higher plasma cortisol levels which interfere with the TSH response to TRH. Another possibility is that it reflects changes in receptor sensitivity and neurotransmitter concentration associated with depression.

Asnis G, Nathan R S, Halbreich, U 1980 TRH tests in depression. Lancet, 1: 424–425
Gold M S, Pottash A, Davies R, Ryan N, Sweeney D, Martin D 1979 Distinguishing unipolar and bipolar depression by thyrotropin release test. Lancet 2: 411–412

275 Acute intermittent porphyria (AIP) is the main variety of these disorders to have psychiatric features in European countries. Psychological symptoms accompany the attack in up to three-quarter of cases and they can be the presenting

features. Histrionic behaviour and emotional instability are the main features, but clouding of consciousness, disorientation and delusions with visual hallucinations can occur. The psychotic manifestations may resemble schizophrenia. In AIP plasma porphobilinogen may be increased and urinary porphobilinogen and d-aminolaevulinic acid are increased during the attack and uroporphyrins will be found in urine that is left to stand or acidified. Faecal coproporphyrin and protoporphyrin excretion is increased. Porphyria variegata, the South African type, may present with either light sensitive skin lesions or in a manner similar to AIP and it is the latter presentation that is occasionally seen in Holland, UK and USA. In this variety urinary porphobilinogen and d-aminolaevulinic acid are increased during attacks and faecal protoporphyrins and coproporphyrins are increased between attacks.

de Grunchy G C 1972 Disorders of pigment metabolism. In: Clinical Haematology in Medical Practice. Blackwell, Oxford
Lishman W A 1978 Endocrine diseases and metabolic disorders. In: Organic Psychiatry. Blackwell, Oxford

276 These are two behavioural techniques used to eliminate maladaptive anxiety related avoidance behaviour patterns. Both procedures involve the presentation of anxiety provoking cues for an extended period of time to a patient who is not allowed to make any avoidance response. Flooding involves exposing the patient *in vivo* to the feared situation in a non-graded manner with no prior effort to reduce the anxiety by alternative means such as drugs. Flooding in imagination is referred to as implosive therapy. The patient is trained in imagination and visualisation skills. Implosion scenes are presented in which the patient is encouraged to experience anxiety symptoms related to the scene. A few long sessions produce a better outcome than the same amount of treatment given over a greater number of short sessions. The patient should stay in contact with the feared object till there are clear indications of definite fear reduction. Theoretically, very short periods of exposure from which the patient escapes while the fear is at its height should increase the avoidance response.

Peck D F, McGuire R J 1988 Behavioural and cognitive approaches. In: Kendell R E, Zealley A K (eds)

Companion to Psychiatric Studies, 4th edn. Churchill Livingstone, Edinburgh

277   This term refers to a disorder of muscle tone in which there is involuntary contraction of skeletal muscles mostly involving the head and neck. Acute dystonia occurs in 2% to 10% of patients who have taken anti-psychotic medication usually within the first few days and is more common in young males. The features consist of intermittent muscular spasms leading to abnormal postures of face and neck, oculogyric crises, blepharospasm, trismus, torticollis and opisthotonos. The acute dystonias are thought to be due to a blockade of dopamine receptors in the nigro-striatal pathway and a relative excess of acetylcholine. The dystonia usually responds to parenteral or oral anticholinergic drugs.

Burke R, Fahn R, Jankovic J, Marsden L, Lang A, Gollomp S, Ilsan J 1982 Tardive dystonia: Late onset and persistent dystonia caused by antipsychotic drugs. Neurology 32: 1335–1346
Silverstone T, Turner P 1982 Drug Treatment in Psychiatry 3rd edn. Routledge & Kegan Paul, London

278   Management consists of prompt recognition of the disorder before a chronic course is established and correction of any upsetting factors at school where appropriate. A careful history from parents and teachers should be elicited and school complaints systematically investigated. Examination of the child should include an assessment of the psychiatric state, physical, social and intellectual development and an important aspect of the evaluation is a school visit. For the child with an acute onset the approach advocated by Kennedy is recommended. This consists of early return to school with firm consistent action involving both of the parents, support from the psychiatric team and liaison with the school. Usually this approach is easily achieved with younger children. Where a longer history prevails, psychotherapeutic approaches may be required in both individual and family based, pharmacological and behavioural treatments. The child is gradually reintroduced to school for short periods at first, accompanied by parents, then with friends until eventually able to enter the classroom alone. The child will need strong support and encouragement

to persue independent activities. Residential treatment may be required for the severely disturbed child. This will allow treatment of the underlying disorder, separation from the family and continued education. Antidepressant medication has been advocated in treatment of school refusal but trials have not confirmed the efficacy of the tricyclic group of drugs.

Berg I 1983 School non-attendance. In: Russell G, Hersov L (eds) Handbook of Psychiatry, 4. The neuroses and personality disorders. Cambridge University Press, Cambridge

Kennedy W A 1965 School phobia: Rapid treatment of fifty cases. Journal of Abnormal psychology 70: 285–289

279 The brain is atrophied and has widened sulci, decreased white matter and ventricular enlargement. Frontal and temporal atrophic changes are more prominent but the parietal and occipital lobes may sometimes be equally affected. The hippocampus and amygdala are usually considerably shrunken. The major microscopic changes are neurofibrillary tangles and plaques in the archi and neocortical regions. Neurofibrillary tangles are helically paired twisted filaments. With the exception of the neocortex, the distribution of tangles is similar to that in old age, but the medial temporal amygdaloid and hippocampal areas are more liable to develop tangles of increased density in Alzheimer's disease. Neocortical tangles are infrequently found in the elderly and their presence is almost always associated with clinical dementia. Senile plaques which contain abnormal nerve cell processes, glial cells and amyloid fibrils develop within the cortical grey matter and occasionally in other brain areas such as the basal ganglia, brain stem and cerebellum. Other minor histological abnormalities include granulovacuolar degeneration, hirano/body formation, neuropil degeneration and vascular or perivascular amyloid degeneration. In contrast to presenile dementia, the pathological diagnosis of senile dementia of Alzheimer's type is more difficult. In the elderly the difference between aging and Alzheimer's disease may be obscured by the presence of age-associated changes such as brain atrophy, neurofibrillary tangles and senile plaques.

Perry R E 1982 The aging brain and its pathology. In: Levy R, Post F (eds) The Psychiatry of Late Life. Blackwell, Oxford

Tomlinson B 1982 Plaques, tangles and Alzheimer's disease. Psychological Medicine 12: 449–459

280 All neuroleptic drugs potentiate the depressant effects of central nervous system depressant drugs. These drugs include alcohol, barbiturates, opiates and benzodiazepines. In the central nervous system anti-psychotics inhibit the effects of stimulants and anorexia inducing medication. They also block the effect of L-Dopa and bromocriptine so reducing their efficacy in Parkinsonism. Lithium, in combination with the phenothiazines may increase the anti-psychotic effects, but may worsen the extrapyramidal effects. The alpha-adrenergic blocking action of the phenothiazines can lead to significant hypotension when combined with other drugs, especially the monoamine-oxidase inhibitors. Chlorpromazine may reverse the anti-hypertensive effect of drugs such as guanethidine and methyldopa. Thioridazine and chlorpromazine have especially strong atropinic properties and combined with the anticholinergic group of drugs may precipitate an atropine psychosis. Drug interactions may occur in the gastrointestinal tract. Colloidal antacids absorb chlorpromazine as well as other drugs administered concurrently. Anticholinergic agents slow gut mobility and enhance intestinal metabolism of chlorpromazine. Antipsychotics inhibit the hepatic metabolism of tricyclic antidepressants and propranolol increasing the plasma levels of these drugs. Interaction with phenytoin has also been described. Phenothiazines, by interfering with glucose metabolism, may necessitate the alteration of antidiabetic dosage regimes.

Salzman C, Hoffman S A 1983 Clinical interaction between psychotropics and other drugs. Hospital Community Psychiatry 34: 897–902
Silverstone T, Turner P 1982 Drug treatment in psychiatry 3rd edn. Routledge & Kegan Paul, London

281 It is a clinical procedure for eliminating anxiety reactions and phobias. Wolpe originally described a three stage approach—relaxation, construction of a hierarchy of fearful situations and presentation of these items from the hierarchy starting with the least threatening stimulus and proceeding in a graded manner. The duration and number of therapy sessions varies depending on the complexity

of the problem and the number of hierarchies to be worked through. Desensitisation may be performed *in vivo* or in fantasy. Occasionally tape recordings, films and group work may be used. With agoraphobic patients desensitisation in fantasy may also be effective particularly if the patient practises at home. Over 66% of patients with phobic disorders show marked improvement with systematic desensitisation and this therapeutic response is still held at nine years follow-up. With simple phobias exposure in fantasy followed by exposure *in vivo* produces marked improvement in over 90% of patients. Desensitisation is also used with other techniques in treating social phobias.

Barlow D H 1980 Behaviour therapy: The next decade. Behaviour Therapy II 315–328
Peck D F, McGuire R J 1988 Behavioural and cognitive therapies. In: Kendell R E, Zealley A K (eds) Companion to Psychiatric Studies, 4th edn. Churchill Livingstone, Edinburgh

282   Three different syndromes can be identified in association with hypoglycaemia. Acute hypoglycaemia occurring in response to an overdose of insulin or hypoglycaemic drugs can present with malaise, anxiety and panic attacks. Feelings of hunger, palpitations, restlessness, tremor, flushing and ataxic gait will also feature. Brief episodes of unconsciousness will culminate in coma in severe cases. An epileptic fit is occasionally the mode of presentation and less commonly focal neurological disturbances such as diplopia, dysphasia or hemiparesis may occur. The subacute syndrome is also episodic and is more usually associated with an insulinoma. The main features of this syndrome are clumsiness and uncharacteristic behaviour such as aggressiveness and disinhibition. Others can become withdrawn and listless with slurred speech and somnolence. Disorientation is usually evident and the patient is frequently unaware of the degree of disability. The chronic form of the syndrome is rare and is almost always due to an insulinoma. It develops insidiously with signs of personality change and emotional lability. Later, memory and intellectual deterioration proceed to a full blown dementia. This insidious decline may be punctuated by symptoms of acute hypoglycaemia.

Lishman W A 1978 Endocrine diseases and metabolic disorders. In: Organic Psychiatry. Blackwell, Oxford

Marks V, Rose F C 1965 Hypoglycaemia. Blackwell, Oxford

283 Patients with affective disorders frequently have abnormal premorbid personality traits but they are not specific to this diagnostic group. Unipolar depressives generally exhibit a 'melancholic personality type' and show features of introversion, lack of confidence, pessimism, unassertiveness, dependency and obsessionality. Unipolar manics tend to have a 'manic personality type' characterised by a tendency to be work orientated, driven, obsessional, extrovert and cyclothymic. A combination of both personality types, as encountered in the majority of bipolar manic depressive patients, generally results in an unremarkable personality make-up, although some have a cyclothymic personality. The question of where personality ends and illness begins has been highlighted by the description of the 'sub-affective disorders'. Akiskal has identified a hyperthymic or 'chronic' hypomanic disorder, a pure cyclothymic with alternating 'highs' and 'lows', a predominantly depressed cyclothymic and a sub-affective dysthymia type with chronic sub-syndrome depressive symptoms which occasionally reach caseness.

Akiskal H S, Hirschfeld R M A, Yerevanian B I 1983 The relationship of personality to affective disorder. Archives of General Psychiatry 40: 801–810

Zerssen D V 1982 Personality and affective disorders. In: Handbook of Affective Disorders. Churchill Livingstone, Edinburgh

284 Bowlby's affectionless psychopathy is the paradigm of the syndrome but, due to improvements in institutions caring for children, it is rarely seen in its entirety. Emotional deprivation may occur in the absence of other forms of deprivation such as lack of intellectual stimulation or inadequate material circumstances. Few children present with the complete picture but many show characteristics such as disinhibited overfriendliness, attention seeking and clinging behaviour and an impaired ability to relate to peers. Frequently some antisocial symptoms such as lying and aggression co-exist.

Rutter M 1981 Maternal deprivation re-assessed. Penguin Books, London

Wolkind S, Rutter M 1985 Separation, loss and
   family relationships. In: Rutter M, Hersov L (eds)
   Child and Adolescent Psychiatry Modern
   Approaches. Blackwell, Oxford

285   Perseveration is the senseless repetition of a goal-
      directed activity after the need for this activity has
      ceased. It can affect all forms of responses, simple
      movements, co-ordinated actions and posture, but
      is seen at its most obvious when speech is
      affected. The patient is unable to get beyond a
      word or phrase which he goes on repeating and
      may repeat in reply to another question. Special
      varieties of perseveration include palilalia and
      logoclonia. In palilalia the perseverated word is
      repeated with increasing frequency while in logo-
      clonia the last syllable of the last word is repeated.
      Stereotypies are regularly repetitive, non-goal
      directed movements such as bodyrocking or foot
      tapping. Perseveration differs from stereotypies in
      that it is initiated by a goal directed activity. The
      word, phrase or idea persists beyond the point at
      which it is relevant in perseveration while in
      stereotypy the same word or phrase is used regard-
      less of the situation.

      Fish F J (ed) 1984 Fish's schizophrenia, 3rd edn.
         Hamilton H Wright, Bristol

286   It is characterised by a delusion of infidelity
      regarding the sexual partner and is also known as
      'the erotic jealousy syndrome', 'psychotic jealousy'
      and the 'morbid jealousy syndrome'. The delusion
      can occur in isolation, but it is often part of
      another psychosis, such as a paranoid state, or can
      occur in association with manic-depressive
      psychosis, schizophrenia, epilepsy, dementia and
      alcoholism. It usually presents in the fourth
      decade and usually starts quite suddenly with the
      subject accusing their partner of infidelity. The
      facts are usually distorted by the patient, past
      events are frequently misinterpreted and they
      often present contradictory evidence or ignore
      facts that would refute their claims. Frequent
      interrogation by the patient may force the spouse
      to make a false confession in the hope of ending
      the matter, but it makes the situation worse. Viol-
      ence is often part of the syndrome and this makes
      it a particularly serious problem as the outcome
      can be fatal. The jealousy is thought to be a
      projection of the patient's own sense of inad-

equacy onto the spouse and this sense of inferiority may be related to a change in financial or social standing, impotence, the patient's own unfaithfulness, homosexuality or an inability to love the spouse.

Enoch D M, Trethowan W H 1979 The Othello syndrome. In: Uncommon Psychiatric Syndromes. Wright, Bristol
Shepherd M 1961 Morbid jealousy. Journal of Medical Science 107: 687–753

287 Psychosurgical procedures are generally directed to the limbic system and bimedial leucotomy has replaced the earlier prefrontal leucotomy or lobotomy. However, other areas of the brain have been operated on, including the hypothalamus, hippocampus, cingulum bundle and the corpus collosum. British neurosurgeons tend to favour the subcaudate area and the medical quadrants of the frontal lobes where subcaudate tractotomies and limbic leucotomies are carried out respectively. All of these operations are now performed with the help of stereotactic instruments which, along with electrode stimulation, enable specific brain areas to be more accurately located.

Bridges P K, Goktepe E D, Maratos J 1973 A comparative review of patients with obsessional neurosis and depression treated by psychosurgery. British Journal of Psychiatry 123: 663–674
Kelly D 1976 Psychosurgery in the 1970s. British Journal of Hospital Medicine 4: 165–174

288 While there is considerable uncertainty about how best to treat bulimia, general management guidelines consist of establishing a working relationship with the patient, interrupting the cycle of binging, vomiting and purging and preventing relapse. Treatment can be conducted on an out-patient basis but in-patient management may be required if the bulimic behaviour is poorly controlled, if the patient is not responding on an out-patient basis or is exhibiting suicidal intent. A variety of psychotherapeutic approaches have been described and they may be supportive or analytic, individual, group or family based. Fairburn has described a cognitive behavioural approach which seems relatively effective in the short term, but long term results remain uncertain. The first stage is designed to interrupt the binging/vomiting cycle and consists of patient education, advice or

weighing, prescribing specific eating patterns and focusing on alternative behaviour. The second stage involves identification of specific stressful situations associated with binging, modification of abnormal attitudes about food, eating and body shape, problem solving training and introducing avoided foods. The final stage centres on planning strategies to address potential relapse. Self-help groups may be of some benefit. There is no role for drugs unless there is a co-existing depressive illness.

Fairburn C 1988 Eating disorders. In: Kendell R E, Zealley A K (eds) Companion to Psychiatric Studies, 4th edn. Churchill Livingstone, Edinburgh

Fairburn C G 1983 Bulimia: its epidemiology and management. In: Stunkard A J, Sellers E (eds) Eating and Its Disorders. New York Press

289 A clear link has been established between anti-social personality in adults and childhood conduct disorders in that the former is almost always preceded by the latter, while only a minority of the conduct disordered children become antisocial adults. Again, drawing from Robins' longitudinal studies, schizophrenic patients, when young, tend to display neurotic symptoms, difficulties with social relationships and antisocial behaviour in the home. While childhood emotional disorders have a good prognosis, adults with neurotic symptoms who have had a childhood disorder will have had an emotional as children. Some continuity also exists between school phobia and agoraphobia, in that 5% of hospitalised school phobics develop agoraphobia as adults. Depressive symptoms in children do not usuallly predict adult depression. However, one study found that 70% of children with a major depressive disorder had a recurrence within five years. Manic-depressive illness, which hardly ever occurs before puberty is likely to re-cur in later life.

Robins L 1978 Study of childhood predictors of adult antisocial behaviour. Psychological Medicine 8: 611–622

Rutter M 1986 Psychopathology and development: Links between childhood and adult life. In: Child and Adolescent Psychiatry. Modern approaches, 2nd edn. Blackwell, Oxford

290 This is a rare syndrome characterised by repeated admission to general hospitals for self-induced or

fictitious symptoms. Such patients will often discharge themselves against medical advice following an argument in the days following surgery, or when they are discovered to have attended and deceived doctors at other hospitals. While 'abdominal', 'haemorrhagic' and 'neurological' forms have been described, an infinite array of presenting symptoms are possible. They are usually self-referred, are admitted through casualty in an acutely distressed state and submit to repeated investigations and surgery. When not in hospital they are frequently in police custody for petty larceny. The syndrome is considered to be related to a life long habit of attention seeking behaviour and the hospital environment is thought to cater for their dependency and narcissistic needs. Others have well marked psychopathic personality traits.

O'Shea B, McGennis A, Cahill A, Falvey A 1984 Munchausen's syndrome. British Journal of Hospital Medicine 31: 269–274

Roy A 1986 Self destructive behaviour. In: Hill P, Murray R, Thorley A (eds) Essentials of Postgraduate Psychiatry 2nd edn. Grune and Stratton, London

291 This syndrome is characterised by mental retardation, physical characteristics such as macroorchidism, prominent ears, prognathism and impaired speech and a fragile site on the X chromosome. Almost all males with this syndrome are mentally retarded. The penis is normal in size and there is no evidence of precocious puberty. Hormonal studies and testicular histology are normal. Patients with this syndrome have a fragile site at the terminus of the long arm of the X chromosome (Xq27). This fragility is revealed when blood lymphocytes are cultured in a medium deficient in folic acid. It has been estimated that the fragile X syndrome may account for up to 30% of X linked mental retardation in males and approximately 10% of all mild mental retardation in females. Herbst and Millar found a frequency of 1.83 per 1,000 males in the general population and calculated a carrier rate of 2.5 per 1,000 for females.

Herbst M, Miller J R 1980 Non-specific X-linked mental retardation II. The frequency in British Columbia. American Journal Medical Genetics 7: 461–469

Nelson Textbook of Paediatrics 1983 12th edn. (eds)
Vaughan V, McKay R, Behrmann R. Saunders,
London

292   The features of this syndrome as described by
Edwards and Gross involve behavioural, subjective and psychophysiological changes, with
impaired control over drinking being a major
aspect. The changes in behaviour focus on the
drinking activities of the dependent person, with
narrowing of the drinking repertoire and salience
of drinking over other activities. The dependent
person reports a subjective awareness of a compulsion to drink, impaired control over his drinking,
combined with a craving for and preoccupation
with alcohol. The psychobiological changes
include development of tolerance, repeated withdrawal symptoms, relief of these symptoms by
further drinking and reinstatement after abstinence.

Edwards G, Gross M M 1976 Alcohol dependence:
provisional description of a clinical syndrome.
British Medical Journal 1: 1058–1061
Murray R 1986 Alcoholism. In: Hill P, Murray R,
Thorley A (eds) Essentials of Postgraduate
Psychiatry 2nd edn. Grune and Stratton, London

293   Psychiatric morbidity is present in some 50% of
cases of Cushing's disease and depression is
undoubtedly the most common psychiatric
symptom. Paranoid features are frequent and in
the more severe forms marked psychomotor
retardation can occur. Emotional lability, restlessness, anxiety and hyperactivity are other features
of this non-specific symptom cluster. Elevated
mood is characteristically associated with therapeutic steroids and the incidence of severe mental
symptoms is only one-third of that associated with
Cushing's disease. The sense of wellbeing associated with steroid treatment can progress, in
predisposed individuals, to a full blown manic
attack. Not infrequently patients treated with
steroids become depressed after the treatment is
withdrawn.

Cohen S I 1982 Psychiatric aspects of Cushing's
syndrome. British Journal of Hospital Medicine
27: 548
Kelly W F, Checkley S A, Bender D A 1980
Cushing's syndrome, tryptophan and depression.
British Journal of Psychiatry 136: 125–132

294   Galactorrhoea, menstrual irregularities or amenorrhoea are commonly observed in patients treated
with neuroleptics and are due to increased levels
of prolactin, probably secondary to suppression of
release of the prolactin-inhibiting factor from the
hypothalamus. Hyperprolactinaemia in men is
associated with decreased libido, impotence and
sterility. Chlorpromazine has a poikilothermic
effect. Improved glucose tolerance may be noted.
There is often a considerable weight gain and
many patients have a markedly increased appetite
and this, with reduced activity resulting from the
sedative effect of the drug, may account for the
weight increase. The syndrome of inappropriate
secretion of antidiuretic hormone can be induced
by anti-psychotic medication. Those patients who
take phenothiazines for many years develop a
slate-grey pigmentation of the skin. Corneal and
lens opacities have also been described and thioridazine in high doses can produce pigmentary
retinopathy.

Silverstone T, Turner P 1982 Drug treatment in
psychiatry, 3rd edn. Routledge & Kegan Paul,
London

295   Distinctions can be made on clinical, genetic and
pathological grounds. Clinically in Pick's disease,
personality changes are noted from the onset,
whereas memory is relatively well preserved. The
euphoria, emotional blunting and aspontaneity of
Pick's disease is contrasted by the depression,
anxiety and catastrophic reactions seen in
Alzheimer's disease. Parietal lobe signs of apraxia,
agnosia and dysgraphia are relatively absent in
Pick's disease, indicating the integrity of the
parietal lobes. Epileptic seizures are more
common in Alzheimer's disease, as are clearly
psychotic manifestations. Hyperalgesia and early
incontinence may be helpful identifying features
of Pick's disease. Differentiation on clinical
grounds is more easily made in the earlier stages
of the illnesses, since ultimately any differences
become submerged. Transmission by dominant
inheritance is claimed for Pick's disease and
whereas most of the cases arise sporadically in
Alzheimer's disease, a slight familial tendency
with a multi-factorial mode of inheritance has
been noted. The pathology of Alzheimer's disease
is one of global cortical atrophy, silver staining
plaques and neurofibrillary tangles. Pick's disease

characteristically affects frontal and temporal lobes with loss of nerve cells, ballooning of cells and plaques and neurofibrillary tangles are absent. In many cases, the true diagnosis is only revealed at autopsy.

Bond M R 1988 Organic disorders. In: Kendell R E, Zealley A K (eds) Companion to Psychiatric Studies, 4th edn. Churchill Livingstone, Edinburgh

296 This controversial condition applies to the serious sequelae that appears to follow repeated mild head injury and has been extensively described in boxers. The amount of damage is proportional to the number and strength of the concussion blows inflicted. Early neurological features include dysarthria, poverty and clumsiness of movement, rigidity, a Parkinsonian-type gait and tremor. Evidence of asymmetrical pyramidal lesions are common from an early stage. In its fully developed form the syndrome consists of pyramidal, extrapyramidal and cerebellar features, along with varying degrees of intellectual and personality changes. Mild memory impairment may progress to severe dementia. Personality changes may include morbid jealousy,' rage reactions, irritability, apathy and paranoid reactions. Occasionally psychotic features may be present. Post mortem examination shows nerve cell loss, neurofibrillary tangles, brain stem damage, cortical infarcts, haemorrhages and characteristically perforation of the septum pellucidum.

Lishman W A 1978 Head injury. In: Organic Psychiatry. Blackwell, Oxford
Roberts A H 1969 Brain damage in boxers. Pitman, London

297 This is a behavioural approach used in treatment of sexual deviation. The technique involves pairing mental images of heterosexual behaviour with a state of sexual arousal. The subject is asked to use his deviant sexual fantasy during masturbation and to switch his deviant fantasy to a heterosexual fantasy just before orgasm. Subsequently, the heterosexual fantasy is introduced earlier and earlier in the sequence. The procedure is based very loosely on the model of classical conditioning. Difficulties are encountered with the timing of stimuli and with voluntary inhibition of responses. A variant of this method borrows the

ideas of 'shaping' and 'fading' from operant conditioning in which the patient is encouraged to change gradually the nature of his deviant fantasies, bringing them gradually nearer to a fantasy of heterosexual intercourse. Despite its widespread use, there is no convincing evidence that this behavioural method is effective in treating homosexuality or other sexual disorders.

Bancroft J 1983 Human sexuality and its problems. Churchill Livingstone, Edinburgh

298 Evidence of psychiatric symptoms can be found in about two-thirds of patients with hypercalcaemia and in a minority of cases they may be the presenting symptoms or dominate the clinical picture. The most common symptoms are depression and fatigue. The onset, which is usually insidious, seems related to the rate of rise in the serum calcium concentration and is so gradual that it may be misdiagnosed as a depression for a number of years. Tension, irritability and explosive outbursts sometimes accompany the depression. Cerebral organic symptoms are found in about 12% of cases and they typically take the form of memory impairment and general mental slowing. These more chronic features may develop into an acute cerebral reaction with disorientation, paranoid delusions, visual hallucinations and aggressive behaviour. With marked hypercalcaemia a stuporose state will supervene and may lead to coma. Recurring convulsions are also occasionally seen.

Petersen P 1968 Psychiatric disorders in primary hyperparathyroidism. Journal of Clinical Endocrinology and Metabolism 28: 1491–1495

299 Treatment depends on the degree of toxicity and this is assessed by the serum lithium concentration and the subject's physical status. Management involves bringing about a rapid reduction in plasma lithium concentration and taking corrective measures for any changes in blood pressure, kidney, cardiac or pulmonary function. Toxicity is usually clinically evident with plasma lithium levels above 1.5 to 2.0 m.mols/litre, but the patient may still have toxic effects when the level has fallen below 1.5 m.mols/litre due to the high tissue concentration of lithium. Treatment for

mild toxicity, that is for levels below 3.0 m.mols/litre, involves ensuring adequate hydration and diuresis and this is probably best managed with an intravenous saline infusion as the patient will usually be unable to take fluids by mouth. If the patient's clinical condition deteriorates, if abnormalities in fluid and electrolytes are not readily corrected, if renal function tests continue to decline or if the serum lithium does not fall by 20% every six hours haemodialysis should be instituted. Those with plasma lithium level greater than 3.0 m.mols/litre at the outset should have haemodialysis and levels greater than 5.0 m.mols/litre have life threatening implications. After the acute phase of the toxicity has subsided the renal, neurological and thyroid function should be assessed.

Schou M 1980 The recognition and management of lithium toxicity. In: Johnson F N (ed) Handbook of Lithium Therapy. MTP Press, Lancaster

300 Tardive dyskinesia is manifested by a wide variety of involuntary movements including oro-lingual dyskinesia, chorea, athetosis, dystonia, tics and facial grimacing. The most common early signs are sucking, chewing, smacking and other signs of the bucco-lingual masticatory syndrome such as tongue protrusion and grimacing. The hands and feet are frequently affected. Movements of the whole trunk such as body rocking, shoulder shrugging, back arching and pelvic gyrations have been described. Dysarthria, dysphagia and dyspnoea are late signs. The syndrome can occur at any stage, even in children, but it is more common in elderly females with diffuse brain damage. Disorders to be considered in the differential diagnosis include schizophrenic stereotyped movements, reversible neuroleptic syndromes, dyskinesias induced by other drugs and neurological disorders that produce involuntary movements such as Parkinsonism, Wilson's disease, Huntington's chorea. When the disorder is associated with anti-psychotic medication it usually begins after several months or years of treatment. The prevalence of tardive dyskinesia has been estimated to range from 5% to 56% of patients treated with long term neuroleptics. The onset is typically insidious and usually occurs while the patient is receiving anti-psychotic medication. It is frequently observed for the first time following

reduction or discontinuation of neuroleptic treatment.

Baldessarini R J, Cole T O, Davis J M, Simpson G, Tarsy D 1980 Tardive dyskinesia: Summary of a task force report of the American Psychiatric Association. American Journal of Psychiatry 137: 1163–1172

Tarsy D 1983 History and definition of tardive dyskinesia. Clinical Neuropharmacology 6: 91–100

301 All the main aspects of pharmacokinetics are altered in the elderly—the rate of absorption, distribution, plasma protein binding, metabolism and excretion. Absorption is reduced due to reduction in blood flow and rate of gastric secretion. The albumin level falls with age and to a greater extent if the elderly person is ill. Decreased serum albumin results in less drug binding sites. Competition for these sites by two highly protein bound drugs may also cause problems. In the elderly the proportion of body fat is modified causing drugs which are lipid soluble, like diazepam, to have a much greater distribution. This is the main reason for the increased half-life of benzodiazepines in the elderly. Old age brings a reduction in liver metabolising activity and renal excreting ability. Hydroxylation and demethylation are usually slower in the elderly, while conjugating processes are little changed. Studies have shown that renal function declines to about 60% of that in younger age groups. Tubular secretion also declines with age. Changes in the cerebral circulation associated with increasing age may also contribute to the differences in response to centrally acting drugs seen in elderly patients.

Cayley A 1985 Drug prescribing in the elderly. British Journal of Hospital Medicine 34(6): 355–358

Silverstone T, Turner P (eds) 1982 Drug treatment in psychiatry. Routledge & Kegan Paul, London

302 Management should probably involve giving the bereaved relative an opportunity to talk through the death with the attending doctor, ensuring that the person has somebody to help him make day to day decisions, as the bereaved are frequently indecisive and ensuring that the patient does not make major changes in his life in the weeks following the death. The patient should be

advised of the tendency towards drug and alcohol abuse at this time, but the short term use of a hypnotic can be useful. Patients who develop psychiatric disorders following a death should have the primary symptoms treated in their own right and not simply managed as an extended form of grief reaction. The usual approach to managing grief reaction is to encourage the person to express his sense of loss and other painful feelings in the belief that if he does not voice his grief he is likely to develop a prolonged bereavement reaction. While surveys of the bereaved indicate that the majority found talking about the death helpful, there is no evidence to suggest that it limits the duration or severity of the grief. So minimal expression of grief should not necessarily be regarded as abnormal.

Clayton P J 1982 Bereavement. In: Paykel E S (ed) Handbook of Affective Disorders. Churchill Livingstone, Edinburgh

303   This is a structured and controlled environment in which the basic principles of learning, such as reinforcement, extinction and punishment are employed to produce behavioural change. The aim of treatment is usually to modify social behaviour through discouraging socially unacceptable actions whilst encouraging those which are adaptive. Token economies share the following characteristics: target behaviours are selected, a system of assessing and monitoring progress is devised and a token or exchange unit is presented to the patient if the desired behaviour is manifest. These tokens can be spent on back up reinforcers which are generally consumable items, visiting privileges or access to recreational activities. Adequately trained staff are essential in implementing and maintaining an effective system. Problems may arise with patient-staff communications, ethical difficulties, maintaining staff and patient morale and recording token transactions. Token economies have been used in many situations, particularly with long stay in-patient populations, retarded children, delinquent children and adults, emotionally disturbed children and children in the normal classroom setting.

Baker R, Hall J N, Hutchinson K, Bridge G 1977. Symptom changes in chronic schizophrenia patients on a token economy: A controlled experiment. British Journal of Psychiatry 131: 381–393

Gelder M G 1983 Behaviour therapy. In: Russell G,
Hersov L (eds) Handbook of Psychiatry 4. The
neuroses and personality disorders. Cambridge
University Press, Cambridge

304 Bouts of intense anxiety with fear of impending
death are the most common mental symptoms and
these may be followed by excitement and confusion after the episode. Attacks are precipitated
by physical exertion, change in posture, raised
intra abdominal pressure, excitement or a shock.
Patients usually present with episodes of palpitations, flushing or blanching, sweating, tremulous-
ness, dizziness, nausea and vomiting. Hypertension
is usually present during the attack and in 80%
of cases between attacks. Hypertensive complications such as angina, heart failure, cerebrovascular accident and epileptic convulsions are not
uncommon.

Lishman W A 1978 Endocrine diseases and metabolic
disorders, Chapter 11. In: Organic Psychiatry.
Blackwell, Oxford

305 Delusions are fixed false beliefs which are out of
keeping with the patient's social and cultural
background and are held with absolute conviction.
Their content is often fantastic or morbid and
they are usually experienced as being of immense
personal significance. Primary or autochthonous
delusions appear de novo or may appear against
a background of a delusional mood. In this delusional mood the person is aware that something
strange is happening; the patient then realises the
meaning of this feeling with a complete delusional
understanding. Schneider claims that delusional
perception is diagnostic of schizophrenia and
claims that the two-membered nature of the delusional perception is important. In delusional
percepiton, he considers that, there is a link from
the patient to the perception and a second link
from the normal perception to the unusual significance. Secondary delusions arise in an understandable way from other psychic events.
Examples of these delusions include those of
persecution, grandeur, nihilism, jealousy, love, ill-
health, poverty and guilt. Their origins can be
traced to affects, drives or morbid personal experiences—for example, a depressive mood swing
may be followed by delusions of guilt, poverty or

nihilism. These delusions may occur in many psychiatric disorders such as schizophrenia, manic and depressive states, drug and alcohol abuse, and in a variety of organic brain disorders.

Hamilton M (ed) 1978 Fish's Clinical
  Psychopathology, 3rd edn. Wright, Bristol

306   Costello, in a review of 11,000 patients, showed that one year after treatment 1% had died, 53% had a continuing drink problem, 25% had no current drinking problems and 21% were lost to follow-up. He concluded that best results were obtained in those patients who were well motivated, received intensive therapy and adequate follow-up. The Rand report, which is an account of a prospective study at 45 treatment centres in the USA, found that while 50% of untreated patients had improved over eighteen months, 70% of those treated showed improvement. This greater improvement was not attributable to any particular treatment method. At 4 year follow-up 15% had died and of the survivors 28% had abstained for the previous six months, 18% were drinking in an asymptomatic way, while 54% had problems with control and were symptomatic. Davies and colleagues concluded that adequate treatment of whatever form was no better than simple 'advice' after they studied 100 male alcoholics, half of whom were randomly assigned to an intensive treatment programme, while the other half received advice only: after one year the outcome in both groups was similar. Vaillant and Milofsky studied untreated alcoholics and showed that at forty-seven years of age 50% were asymptomatic drinkers or abstinent. Outcome was related to good motivation, a supportive family, health and social competence and progress at six months was found to be a valuable predictor of longer term prognosis.

Armour D, Polich J, Stanbul H 1976 Alcoholism and
  treatment. National Institute of Alcohol Abuse and
  Alcoholism. The Rank Corporation, Santa Monica,
  California.
Cutting J 1979 Alcohol dependence and alcohol-
  related disabilities. In: Granville-Grossman K (ed)
  Recent Advances in Clinical Psychiatry 3. Churchill
  Livingstone, Edinburgh
Vaillant G, Milofsky E S 1982 Natural history of
  male alcoholism IV. Paths to recovery. Archives of
  General Psychiatry 39: 127–133

307 Hypogonadism and other organic disorders are the main indications for drug therapy in sexual dysfunction, their value for psychologically based disorders being very limited. Androgen replacement therapy usually improves sexual interest and ejaculatory function in hypogonadal men where low levels of testosterone are demonstrated. Recent evidence suggests that testosterone therapy may help sexual interest even when circulating levels of testosterone are normal. Androgen replacement therapy usually restores erectile function with hypogonadism, though it is unclear whether the erectile dysfunction is caused directly by hypogonadism. Bromocriptine is of value in erectile dysfunction if it is associated with hyperprolactinaemia. Several drug therapies have been tried to treat premature ejaculation. These include thioridazine, monoamine oxidase inhibitors and clomipramine. However, because premature ejaculation usually responds well to behavioural techniques and nearly always has a psychogenic basis, the use of these drugs is probably unjustified. Androgen therapy may have a role in treatment of women whose sexual interest has decreased following oophorectomy or the menopause. Oestrogen therapy may also improve sexual interest in post-menopausal women and help prevent genital atrophic changes, though the risk of it inducing uterine carcinoma must be considered.

Hawton K 1985 Sexual dysfunction. British Journal of Hospital Medicine 34(4): 207–209
O'Carroll R, Bancroft J 1984 Testosterone therapy for low sexual interest and erectile dysfunction in men: A controlled study. British Journal of Psychiatry 145: 146–152

308 Problem drinkers will present in different ways to the different treatment facilities. Alcohol abuse is found to be a significant factor in a large proportion of general hospital patients. Nolan judged alcoholism to be a significant factor in 14% of patients while Moser reported up to 45% of general hospital patients were alcoholic. The alcohol related disorders include hepatic cirrhosis, gastritis, peptic ulceration, pancreatitis, cardiomyopathies, tuberculosis and peripheral neuropathy. Psychiatric disorders which may be significantly associated with excess alcohol include depressive states, mania, Wernicke-Korsakoff's

syndrome, intellectual impairment, sexual problems and suicide. The family doctor is uniquely placed to detect problem drinkers. Factors considered to indicate those 'at risk' include those patients who smell of alcohol at the consultation, those with a positive family history, single men over forty, need for repeated sick notes on Mondays, alcohol related physical and psychiatric disorders, marital disharmony and behavioural problems in children. Emergency services may detect the problem drinker as these people have an increased incidence of accidents at home, in work and on the road. Accidents at home and at work are increased threefold and in excess of one-third of drivers killed in Britain have blood alcohol levels above the statutory limit. Problem drinkers may be noted among those charged with drunken offences, prisoners serving short term sentences and in those people residing in hostels for the destitute. High risk occupational groups include those working in the catering trade, publicans, journalists, entertainers, company executives, doctors and the armed forces.

Moser J 1974 Problems and programmes related to alcohol and drug dependence in 33 countries. World Health Organisation, Geneva Royal College of Psychiatrists 1979 Report of the special committee on alcohol and alcoholism. Tavistock, London
Wilkins T H 1974 The hidden alcoholic in general practice. Elek Science, London

309 Only rarely will uraemia first present to a psychiatrist as the patient, in most instances, looks unwell. The first psychiatric manifestations are progressive anergia and drowsiness and the patient complains of mental and physical fatigue. They often have short periods in which they show normal activity. As the uraemia progresses memory impairment and disorientation occur. While depression and emotional withdrawal are usually marked, agitation and hostility are occasionally seen. These periods of depression and disorientation fluctuate markedly and the patient's mood and cognition can be normal for short periods. Acute delirium occurs in one-third of cases with the usual features of apprehension, disorientation and hallucinations. Reports of functional psychosis occurring in uraemia are probably a reflection of the patient's premorbid personality and inherited predisposition to developing a

211

psychotic state being present, alongside features of a cerebral organic reaction.

Cutting J, McClelland R 1986 Psychiatric manifestations of organic illness. In: Hill P, Murray R, Thorley A (eds) Essentials of Postgraduate Psychiatry 2nd edn. Grune and Stratton, London
Lishman W A 1978 Endocrine diseases and metabolic disorders. In: Organic Psychiatry. Blackwell, Oxford

310 A calm sympathetic interview which will help to delineate the symptoms and simultaneously present a quiet reassuring approach to the patient is the first step. If it is concluded that the symptoms are in keeping with the psychological and somatic complaints of primary anxiety then being able to assure that there is no evidence of a cardiac or other serious medical disorders will often bring significant relief. Listening, allowing the patient to ventilate his emotional concerns and offering realistic psychological support are the main therapeutic approaches in the initial stages. Giving an explanation of the somatic complaints, limiting the tendency to hyperventilate and deep muscle relaxation therapy will frequently limit the extent of an acute anxiety state. For more severe symptoms a minor tranquilliser and/or a beta-adrenergic blocking drug may be necessary so that the patient can attend to the advice and other treatments that are available. Anxiety symptoms which occur as part of another psychiatric disorder should be managed with the same interview and supportive psychotherapeutic techniques while the treatment for the primary disorder is being instituted.

Urbaitis J C 1983 Anxiety. In: Psychiatric Emergencies. Appleton-Century-Crofts, Norwalk, Connecticut

311 Before commencing a plan of treatment a full assessment of the cause, nature and extent of the problem must be sought. Insomnia could be secondary to many disorders such as change in environment, anxiety and fear, psychiatric illness particularly depression, alcohol abuse, pain, drugs or somatic illnesses. One should treat appropriately the underlying cause. General measures include increasing daytime activities, taking hot milk at night time, having structured routines and leaving a light on at night if fear is a factor. The

main categories of drugs available are barbiturates, benzodiazepines and chloralhydrate. Barbiturates are not recommended because of dependency, enzyme induction and toxicity in overdose. Benzodiazepines are safe in overdose, do not cause hepatic enzyme induction but can cause respiratory depression, dependence and tolerance. A benzodiazepine which is quickly absorbed with a short half-life should be selected. It is recommended that a hypnotic drug should only be a temporary measure. Chloralhydrate is a relatively weak hypnotic and its main disadvantages are its unpleasant taste and its tendency to cause gastric irritation. The preparation dichloral phenazone, which is in tablet form, may be particularly useful in the elderly.

Oswald I 1988 Sleep disorders. In: Kendell R E, Zealley A K (eds) Companion to Psychiatric Studies, 4th edn. Churchill Livingstone, Edinburgh

312 The original concept of endogenous depression still has widespread support. A large series of factor and cluster analytic studies have identified a set of characteristic features such as early morning wakening, psychomotor retardation or agitation, distinct quality of mood, weight loss, impaired concentration, severely depressed mood and inability to respond to improvements in the environment. Pure 'endogenous depression', that is occurring without precipitating life events, is not very common and most clinicians now define this form of depression on the basis of the overall clinical picture, rather than simply by the absence of stressful life events. Endogenous features predict a good response to ECT and tricyclic antidepressants. Failure of the cortisol hypersecretion associated with this form of depression to be suppressed by dexamethasone, a blunted TSH response to intravenous TRH and a shortened REM latency and increased REM density on the sleep EEG are other features associated with endogenous depression. There are no clear differences between endogenous depression and bipolar depression. While the evidence for endogenous depression being a homogenous clinical entity is persuasive, the position of neurotic depression is uncertain and it is likely that it represents a heterogenous collection of syndromes. The term 'neurotic' is often used interchangeably with 'reactive', but the latter refers to an acute onset

depression precipitated by events and is likely to clear up as soon as the situation is resolved. Factor analytic studies of neurotic depressions tend to produce items such as immaturity, histrionic behaviour, inadequacy, responsivity of mood, initial insomnia, self pity, irritability, hypochondriasis and sudden onset in relation to precipitating factors.

Andreasen N C 1982 Concepts, diagnosis and classification, In: Paykel E S (ed) Handbook of Affective Disorders. Churchill Livingstone, Edinburgh

Checkley S 1986 Affective disorder: Depression. In: Hill P, Murray A, Thorley A (eds) Essentials of Postgraduate Psychiatry 2nd ed. Grune and Stratton, London

313　This is an evolving syndrome which appears approximately 6–8 hours after a substantial fall in blood alcohol levels. Early symptoms include restlessness, tremor, increasing irritability, muscle cramps, gastro-intestinal symptoms such as nausea and vomiting, depressed or tearful affect and sleep disturbance. These symptoms progress over the next 24 hours and may advance to include grand mal seizures, autonomic over-activity and confusional state. There is great variability in the severity and duration of the syndrome, with only 5–6% progressing to the most severe manifestions of withdrawl. Delirium tremens becomes manifest only after several days of abstinence and generally follows a history of many weeks or months of chronic intoxication. It is characterised by clouding of consciousness, with disorientation in time and space, impaired concentration, hallucinations which are mainly visual but may be auditory or tractile, illusions and delusions, which are often of a paranoid nature. The patient is usually very agitated, has a coarse irregular tremor, speech is usually slurred and autonomic over-activity is characteristic. The mood and affect are marked by their lability but apprehension and fear are more common. In the majority of cases delirium tremens is of short duration, though sometimes it may show a chronic relapsing course for many weeks. Trauma or infection complicates the presentation in up to 50% of cases. Metabolic abnormalities, cardiovascular problems and Wernicke's encephalopathy may occur concomitantly.

Cutting J 1979 Alcohol dependence and alcohol-related disabilities. In: Granville–Grossman K (ed.) Recent

Advances in Clinical Psychiatry 3. Churchill
Livingstone, Edinburgh
Murray R 1986 Alcoholism. In: Hill P, Murray R,
Thorley A (eds) Essentials of Postgraduate
Psychiatry 2nd edn. Grune and Stratton, London

314 The notion of being possessed, assuming one
accepts that it is related to a disordered mind, may
be seen in psychotic patients where it is a delusion
and in neurotic states where it can either be an
obsession or near delusional hysterical belief.
When present as a delusion the subject is either
in a depressed state or is suffering from paranoid
schizophrenia. In the former the person's sense of
worthlessness is exaggerated to its ultimate degree
and he is convinced that he is involved with the
devil or possessed by an evil spirit. In schizophrenia hallucinatory or passivity experiences may
be attributed to some diabolical agent. Today,
disorders of ego strength are less likely to involve
the devil and more likely to be attributed to
radiowaves, television or computers. Cultural and
personal factors determine the content of the
delusions. In neurotic disorders the idea of being
possessed is thought to result from a mixture of
cultural beliefs and the need to act out aspects of
personal psychodynamics. Freud regarded it as a
form of neurosis where there is a projection of
rejected and repressed impulses into the outer
world.

Enoch D M, Trethowan W H 1979 Possession states
and allied syndromes. In: Uncommon Psychiatric
Syndromes. Wright, Bristol

315 Epileptic seizures are the most common physical
sequelae and they occur following some 2% of
stereotactic operations and after as many as 10%
of non-stereotactic procedures. Overt frontal lobe
syndromes are now extremely rare complications,
while disinhibition or lethargy are said to occur
in 5 to 10% of cases. Complications following
psychosurgery have lessened with advances in
general anaesthesia and surgical procedures and
more particularly because localised operations are
now possible with stereotactic techniques. Other
physical complications include haemorrhage and
infection. The mortality rate for psychosurgery is
between 0% and 0.2%.

Clare A 1979 Psychosurgery and electroconvulsive
therapy. In: Hill P, Murray R, Thorley A (eds)

Essentials of Postgraduate Psychiatry 1st edn.
Academic Press, London

Goktepe E D, Young L G, Bridges P K 1975 A
further review of stereotactic subcaudate tractotomy.
British Journal of Psychiatry 126: 270–280

316 Epidemiological findings suggest that socio-cultural factors contribute to the development of anorexia nervosa. It affects predominantly middle and upper class teenage girls in developed countries. Although relatively rare in developing countries, when identified it is associated with urbanised ethnic groups from upper social classes. The ideals for feminine beauty have become notably thinner and Garner demonstrated a significant reduction in measurements in Playboy centrefold girls. The enormous pressure on women to meet the current thinner standard for their physical attractiveness has provided a growing impetus for dieting. Media and the fashion industry probably encourage the association of the thin image with positive attributes such as success, beauty, confidence and happiness. This has occurred within the context of changing social, sexual and vocational role expectations for women. That such pressure may precipitate the development of anorexia nervosa seems to be confirmed by the findings that the condition is more common among women whose dieting and weight control are a career requirement, such as ballet dancers, models, athletes and in that there is a real increase in the incidence of the disorder in recent years. Competition would appear to intensify the risk. These examples do not prove that socio-cultural influences specifically cause eating disorders, but rather that they increase the likelihood of their development.

Darby P, Garfinkel P, Garner D, Coscine D (eds)
1981 Anorexia nervosa. Recent developments in
research. Neurology and Neurobiology. Alan R Liss,
New York
Garner D M, Garfinkel P 1980 Sociocultural factors
in the development of anorexia nervosa.
Psychological Medicine 10: 647–656

317 The prevalence rate for a diagnosable psychiatric disorder among teenagers is 15 to 20%. Epidemiological studies suggest that 40% of adolescents with a psychiatric disorder have an affective illness. A similar proportion are conduct disordered and half of these have an unsocialised conduct disorder. A further 20% of the psychiatr-

ically disordered adolescents have a mixed disorder of conduct and emotions. Psychosis is uncommon among younger adolescents where the prevalence rate is 0.1%, but this figure doubles for older teenagers. Psychiatric disorder in adolescence is composed of contributions from child and adult age groups which the teenage years link. During adolescence there is an increase in the rate of depression, suicide, parasuicide, schizophrenia, anorexia nervosa, drug and alcohol dependency, agoraphobia and social phobia, while disorders with a strong developmental component such as faecal soiling, enuresis, hyperkinetic syndrome, tics and separation anxiety become less common.

Graham P, Rutter M 1973 Psychiatric disorder in the young adolescent: A follow up study. Proceedings of the Royal Society of Medicine 66: 1126–1229

Leslie S A 1974 Psychiatric disorder in the young adolescents of an industrial town. British Journal of Psychiatry 125: 113–124

Rutter M (ed) 1979 Changing youth in a changing society. Nuffield Provincial Hospital Trust, London

318 This syndrome is usually evident at birth, when the most striking physical abnormalities are those affecting the face and skull. All of these children are mentally retarded, having an IQ range between 20 and 70. There is usually occipital flattening giving a brachycephalic skull. The neck is short and fontanelles are late to close. Ocular manifestations include mongoloid slant to the palpebral fissures, epicanthic folds, cataracts, brushfield spots in the iris, strabismus and acute keratoconus with corneal hydrop. Eruption of the teeth is frequently delayed and the positioning irregular. Commonly there is a high arched palate with protrusion of the tongue which is normal in size. Their stature is small and they have short limbs and spade-like hands. A transverse palmar crease, the simian crease, occurs in 40% of cases. The fingers may be webbed, shorter than normal and the little finger may be curved inwards. The big toe is generally short and there is a wide space between the first and second toe. Syndactyly of the toes may occur. The dermatoglyphic pattern of the hands and feet is pathognomonic. Cardiac anomalies which occur in up to 20% are chiefly those of ventricular septal defect. Other features include laxity of the joints, cryptorchidism, intestinal atresia and inperforate anus. There is an increased likelihood of developing leukaemia and

lymphocytic thyroiditis occurs in 30% of cases. Senile degenerative brain changes, with dementia occurs at an earlier age than usual.

Nelson Textbook of Paediatrics 1983 '12th edn.
Vaughan V, McKay R, Behrmann R (eds).
Saunders, London

319 Wernicke-Korsakoff's syndrome, alcoholic dementia and peripheral neuropathy are the main neurological sequelae. Cognitive impairment ranges from mild memory impairment, difficulty learning new material, disturbance of visuo-spatial and visuo-perceptive skills as demonstrated on psychometric testing, to gross diffuse brain damage. Computerised tomography have shown evidence of cerebral atrophy in up to 50% of alcoholics. Alcoholic cerebellar degeneration presents as ataxia of stance and gait. Approximately 10% of alcoholics have convulsions and these may be related to acute alcohol intoxication, withdrawal states, hypoglycaemia or cerebral damage. Rare conditions include central pontine myelinolysis, proximal myopathy and primary degeneration of the corpus callosum in the Marchiafava-Bignami syndrome.

Murray R 1986 Alcoholism. In: Hill P, Murray R, Thorley A (eds) Essentials of Postgraduate Psychiatry 2nd edn. Grune and Stratton, London
Ray H A, Acker W, Shaw G K, Lishman W A 1982 Computerised tomography of the brain in chronic alcoholism. Brain 105: 497–514

320 Cognitive and mood disturbance are the two main groupings. Psychiatric morbidity is present in about 75% of cases and intellectual impairment, which is usually mild, is present in about two-thirds of instances. The latter presents as loss of memory for recent events, impaired conceptual thinking and non-verbal reasoning. Dementia ia occasionally encountered. Of the mood disturbances, depression and euphoria are each found in about 25% of cases. Depression, which tends to be an early feature, is considered to be reactive in nature, to be related to the implications of the diagnosis and unrelated to cerebral pathology. Visual disturbance, impotence, loss of sphincter control and ataxia also contribute to the depression. Euphoria presents with a cheerful complacency which is indifferent to the physical disability and tends to correlate with the degree

of intellectual impairment. It is associated with plaque lesions on the frontal lobes. Other features of frontal lobe involvement such as disinhibition, a fatuous manner and emotional lability are seen. The so called personality changes associated with multiple sclerosis probably reflect the initial depression and the later intellectual deterioration, and frontal lobe involvement.

Surridge D 1969 An investigation into some psychiatric aspects of multiple sclerosis. British Journal of Psychiatry 115: 749–764

Whitlock A 1984 Emotional disorder in multiple sclerosis. In: Simons A F (ed) Multiple Sclerosis. Heinemann, London

321 The more commonly encountered causes are alcohol abuse, functional illness, in particular depression, Alzheimer's disease and multi-infarct dementia. Other possible causes would include traumatic subdural haematoma, primary or metastatic carcinoma, alcoholic dementia, Parkinson's disease and endocrine disorders such as hypothyroidism, Addison's and parathyroid disorder. Infrequently memory loss might be as a result of vitamin deficiency, normal pressure hydrocephalus, cranial arteritis, neurosyphilis, sytemic lupus erythematosis, metabolic disorder or hereditary illnesses such as Huntington's Chorea or Wilson's disease. Rarer causes are Pick's disease, Jacob-Creutzfeld disease, punch drunk syndrome and metal toxicity.

Bond M R 1988 Organic disorders. In: Kendell R E, Zealley A K (eds) Companion to Psychiatric Studies, 4th edn. Churchill Livingstone, Edinburgh

322 Childhood suicide is rare. Shaffer (1974), in an eight-year period, found none were younger than twelve years of age and in the ten to fourteen age group he found an incidence of 1:800,000. Successful suicide victims were usually either of above average intelligence or were intellectually retarded. There is a five-fold male predominance and a marked sex difference in methods used; girls favour overdose while boys use violent means such as hanging, or less commonly firearms. Shaffer noted that suicides were not impulsive acts but often showed evidence of very careful planning, one-quarter occurred within two weeks of the child's birthday. A high proportion of victims

were socially isolated and over one-half of them had a first degree relative with a major psychiatric disorder. Two-thirds of the children exhibited antisocial problems, the same proportion showed emotional disturbance and seventeen of thirty children exhibited both forms of disturbance. For one-third a 'disciplinary crisis' appeared as a precipitant and the child's parents were about to be informed of a misdemeanour, such as truanting. At least 40% had told someone of their suicidal ideas beforehand. Most children were living with one or two natural parents at the time of the act and the prevalence of broken homes in this group was, in fact, no higher than in other psychiatrically disturbed children. However, evidence of particular instability may be inferred from the subsequent break up of one in four of the marriages.

Shaffer D 1974 Suicide in childhood or early adolescence. Journal of Child Psychology, Psychiatry 45: 406–451
Shaffer D 1985 Depression, mania and suicidal acts. In: Rutter M, Hersov L (eds) Child and Adolescent Psychiatry 2nd edn. Blackwell, Oxford

323 This condition is characterised by involuntary muscular spasm which results in slow writhing dystonic movements of the head and neck and may be accompanied by a sustained abnormal posture. It commonly starts between the age of 30 and 50 and has an equal sex ratio. The onset is usually gradual but can occur suddenly and is often related to an acute emotional shock. The sternomastoid muscle is usually prominently involved drawing the head laterally and rotating the chin. Sometimes the head may be flexed laterally or pulled forward or backward. In time the muscular spasm comes to be continuous and muscle hypertrophy and cervical spondylosis may result. Occasionally facial grimacing, shoulder shrugging or athetoid movements of the upper limbs are evident. It is not under conscious control, tends to lessen with sleep or when the subject is actively engaged and is exacerbated by stress. The course of spasmodic torticollis is usually one of slow decline over the years, although remission occurs in a quarter of cases. Psychogenic and organic explanations have been forwarded and its resemblance to other basal ganglia syndromes tend to favour an organic causation. Therapeutic approaches have been varied

ranging from behaviour therapy to stereotactic surgery, but best results seem to come from haloperidol. Psychotherapy is useful where the person has an anxious, immature personality.

Cockburn J J 1971 Spasmodic torticollis: A psychogenic condition? Journal of Psychosomatic Response 15: 471–477
Lishman W A 1978 Other disorders affecting the nervous system. In: Organic Psychiatry. Blackwell, Oxford

324   While many men with alcoholism may drink openly, women are inclined to conceal their drinking. Markers of abuse include chronic poor nutrition, self-neglect, inadequate clothing, hypothermia, episodic confusion and restriction of lifestyle. Medical problems which raise the possibility of abuse include liver cirrhosis, confusional states, peripheral neuropathy, ataxia and memory impairment. More commonly, the presenting features are more subtly connected with alcohol. Recurrent fractures or falls, incontinence, tremor, macrocytosis and vitamin deficiencies, violent outbursts, drunkenness and police involvement, defaulting from day care and non-compliance with medication are all clues to abuse. Bereavement, physical disability and retirement have been identified as major precipitants. About one-third of elderly patients with alcohol related problems are drinking as a consequence of a dementing illness; dementia precedes drinking and alcohol causes further confusion and impairment of judgement. Alcohol abuse may also occur in the course of a depressive illness.

Mishara B L, Kastenbaum R 1980 Alcohol and old age. Grune and Stratton, New York
Rosin A J, Glatt M 1971 Alcohol excess in the elderly. Quarterly Journal of Studies in Alcoholism 32: 53–59
Wattis J P 1983 Alcohol and old people. British Journal of Psychiatry 143: 306–307

325   The notion that psychiatric disorders are rare in underdeveloped countries is now known to be untrue. Reported differences in the prevalence rates of the various mental illnesses need to be interpreted cautiously as different concepts of mental illness, diagnostic criteria and treatment facilities will have a bearing on these rates. If clear operational criteria are used, such as those of the

Present State Examination, or the Research Diagnostic Criteria, schizophrenia is found to be equally prevalent in widely different cultures, although the content of delusions will be different. Confusion, excitement and unsystematized delusions are common in the early stages of schizophrenia in illiterate Africans and catatonia is a particularly prominent feature in India. Depressive illnesses, once thought to be rare in the third world, are frequently encountered in these cultures, but feelings of guilt, unworthiness and suicide are not very common features. Paranoid delusions, hypochondriasis, somatic complaints and agitation are reported to occur more frequently than in depressives in Britain. Neurotic disorders have also been described in almost every culture and hysterical conversion and dissociative states are particularly common in underdeveloped countries. Overall, transcultural studies suggest that the major forms of mental illness present with equal frequency in most cultures.

Jablenxky A, Sartorius N 1975 Culture and schizophrenia. Psychological Medicine 5: 113–124
Teja J S, Narang R L, Aggarwal A K 1971 Depression across cultures. British Journal of Psychiatry 119: 253–260

326 The principal features of this syndrome are ocular abnormalities, ataxia of gait and mental confusion. The onset is characteristically acute, with ocular and ataxic signs manifesting before the confusional state. Ocular manifestations include vertical and horizontal nystagmus, lateral rectus palsy and paralysis of conjugate gaze. Ataxia of gait varies in severity ranging from difficulty in standing to minor abnormalities on heel-to-toe walking. Abnormal mental states occur in 90% of patients. Generally the patient shows dullness, apathy, inattention, disorientation and memory derangement. Profound lowering of consciousness is rare. A delirious state with agitation, disorientation and abnormal perceptual phenomena is sometimes seen. A small number of patients remain alert and attentive and show a typical Korsakoff memory defect. As the global confusion recedes memory defects become clearly established. In addition to the classical triad of symptoms, peripheral neuropathy and signs of poor nutrition and vitamin deficiencies are common features. With the administration of thiamine ocular abnormalities show early recovery but horizontal nystagmus may

be a permanent sequel. Ataxia improves within one week of starting treatment but remains incomplete in up to 50% of cases. The global confusion is slow to recover but usually clears completely to leave a short term memory defect.

Lishman W A 1978 Vitamin deficiencies. In: Organic Psychiatry. Blackwell, Oxford

Victor M 1983 Mental disorders due to alcoholism. In: Lader M (ed) Handbook of Psychiatry 2 Mental disorders and somatic illness. Cambridge University Press, Cambridge

327 These are disturbances of sleep lasting 1–2 minutes during which the subject screams or moans, seems to experience intense anxiety and has a rapid pulse and a panting respiration. The person is usually amnesic for the event but may be able to recall a single frightening image. Night terrors and somnambulism often occur in the same individual, they tend to run in families and they are typically experienced by children who tend to grow out of them, or by adult males who have high anxiety levels. Night terrors are distinguished from nightmares in that they arise during stages 3 and 4 of non-REM sleep, while the latter occur during the REM phase. Diazepam may be useful in limiting the phenomenon.

Fisher C, Kahn E, Edwards A, Davis D M 1973 A psycho-physiological study of nightmares and night terrors 1: Physiological aspects of the stage 4 night terror. Journal of Nervous and Mental Disorders 157: 75–98

Kales A, Kales J D 1974 Sleep disorders: Recent findings in the diagnosis and treatment of disturbed sleep. New England Journal of Medicine 290: 487–499

328 This syndrome is characterised by a disturbance of short term memory occurring in clear consciousness. The memory impairment takes the form of inability to learn new information or anterograde amnesia and an inability to remember events covering a period of months to years before the onset of the illness or retrograde amnesia. This retrograde amnesia is often dense but patterns of information may be retained. Remote memory, though impaired, is much better preserved. Long established skills such as speaking, writing or technical skills acquired in the past are unaffected. Immediate memory remains intact. Confabulation, where the patients give a reasonably coherent

but false account of an event, is often described as a characteristic feature of this syndrome, but it is not always present and is not essential to make the diagnosis. There is often difficulty in sustaining mental activity and the patient has difficulty changing from one set task to another. Thinking is often stereotyped, the patient can only construct the simplest concepts and may show difficulties in speed and organisation. These patients tend to be apathetic and show only limited insight. Once the syndrome is established significant improvement occurs in less than 20%. Korsakoff's syndrome is usually the sequel of Wernické encephalopathy.

Lishman W A 1978 Toxic disorders. In: Organic Psychiatry. Blackwell, Oxford

Bond M R 1988 Organic disorders. In: Kendell R E, Zealley A K (eds) Companion to Psychiatric Studies, 4th edn. Churchill Livingstone, Edinburgh

329 This is a genetic disorder of phenylalanine metabolism and mental retardation, usually of a severe degree, is its major manifestation. It occurs in 1 in 14,000 births and is transmitted by an autosomal recessive gene. Brain damage is caused by accumulation of abnormal levels of phenylalanine in the absence of activity of the hepatic enzyme phenylalanine hydroxylase. The untreated child exhibits moderate to severe mental retardation, blond hair, fair skin and blue eyes, a tendency to develop eczema. Many show autistic features such as lack of emotional response but they become unusually attached to small objects. Approximately one-third develop convulsions, usually of grand mal type, which disappear with age. The majority show minor EEG abnormalities. The subnormality is not progressive and it seems that the retardation occurs at a particularly sensitive phase of the brain's development. Once established the brain damage is irreversible so that the main purpose of treatment in phenylketonuria is prevention. A diet restricted in phenylalanine is begun as soon after birth since the diagnosis can be established at this stage. The optimum serum level of phenylalanine to be maintained is between 5 and 9 mg/dl. The diet is continued for a variable time into childhood. Over 90% of children born to phenylketonuria mothers who are not on dietary restriction at the time of conception will be mentally retarded with microcephaly and

stunted intrauterine growth. This observation indicates that these women should be identified and a low phenylalanine diet introduced before conception.

Cytryn L, Lourie R S 1981 Mental retardation. In: Kaplan H I, Sadock B S (eds) Modern Synopsis of Comprehensive Textbook of Psychiatry 3rd edn. Williams and Wilkins, Baltimore

330 There is a wide range of tests varying from brief tests used by clinicians which lack adequate standardisation and validity and which may not be particularly useful in distinguishing between organic and functional disorders to detailed tests which are more reliable but too cumbersome for use with every patient. In interpreting psychological tests which indicate brain damage, one must ask whether the subjects concentration was adequate to perform the test, as depression, sustained anxiety or hallucinatory experiences may give scores consistent with brain damage. Clinical tests of orientation and information are useful in identifying brain damage, but the Digit Span test and the Mill Hill Vocabulary score are not reliable. The Weschsler Deterioration Indices are probably the most widely used measures of organic impairment and the performance scores are more susceptible to change. A discrepancy of greater than 20 points between the verbal and performance scores is a statistically significant indication of organic impairment and is a useful guide when interpreted in the light of the subjects mental state and other psychological measures of brain damage. Verbal learning abilities which are significantly impaired by brain damage can be tested by the Modified Word Learning Test and the Paired Associate Learning Test. Other tests help to localise the site of the damage; a WAIS Performance score which is greater than the verbal IQ characterise left hemisphere damage and the Halstead Category Test and the Rey Osterreth Test are particularly sensitive to frontal and right temporal lesions respectively.

Cutting J, McClelland R 1986 Psychiatric manifestations of organic illness. In: Hill P, Murray R, Thorley A (eds) Essentials of Postgraduate Psychiatry 2nd edn. Grune and Stratton, London
Hinton J, Withers E 1971 The usefulness of clinical tests of sensorium. British Journal of Psychology 119: 9–18

331 The most significant differences between Type I and II is the selective severity of loss of sub-cortical cells in Alzheimer's Type II. In Type II, the early onset form, senile plaques and neurofibrillary tangles are present in abundance. Significant outfall of neurones occurs in the temporal, frontal and cingulate gyri, the locus coeruleus and the basal neucleus of Meynert. In Type I or the late onset form, senile plaques and neurofibrillary tangles are found in the cortex and hippocampus but no significant difference is found between late onset and controls with regard to outfall of neurones. In Type II choline acetyltransferase activity is reduced in the temporal lobe and a decline in serotonin is observed. Diminution of choline acetyltransferase activity is more extensive iin the early onset type, both in the temporal and frontal lobes but it is confined to the temporal lobes in Type I. Noradrenaline shows a significant decline in the frontal, temporal and cinqulate gyri, but no significant decline is observed in the late onset variety. Gamma-aminobutyric acid and somatostatin also shows a significant decline in Type II. Serotonin activity declines in both early and late types.

Rosser M, Iverson L, Reynolds G, Mountjoy C, Roth M 1984 Neurochemical characteristics of early and late onset types of Alzheimer's disease. British Medical Journal 288: 961–964

332 This syndrome, which was first described in South-East Asia but which is not confined to that region, is characterised by a prodromal period of depressive withdrawal followed by aggressive outbursts in which the individual violently attacks people, animals or objects. Homicide is a common outcome and the person frequently kills himself or is killed in the physical turmoil. At the end of the bout the person is usually exhausted and has little memory of the event. Before the middle of the nineteenth century Amok was considered to be an acceptable response of an individual who was being unfairly treated by society. It is now considered to be a socially unacceptable and unnecessary mode of behaviour and is recognised to be a form of hysterical dissociative state which can be of primary origin or occur in the course of a chronic mental disorder.

Lloyd G, Bebbington P 1986 Social and transcultural psychiatry. In: Hill P, Murray R, Thorley A (eds)

Essentials of Postgraduate Psychiatry 2nd edn.
Grune and Stratton, London

333   Disulfiram and alcohol interact to produce unpleasant symptoms and for this reason disulfiram is prescribed as a deterrent against further drinking. When taken with alcohol it produces an acetaldehyde mediated aversive reaction and the syndrome so produced is characterised by facial flushing, widespread vasodilation, dyspnoea, nausea, hypotension and tachycardia. Occasionally cardiac arrhythmias and severe hypotension occurs and fatalities have been described. The reaction is thought to be due to an accumulation of acetaldehyde and a release of histamine. The drug is only prescribed for those willing to comply and who are aware of the potential toxicity. Well motivated patients who are intent on remaining abstinent find it a useful personal deterrent. The efficacy of disulfiram is uncertain. Common side-effects include fatigue, halitosis and nausea and depression, psychotic states, impotence and peripheral neuropathy are occasionally encountered.

Madden J S 1979 A guide to alcohol and drug
    dependence. Wright, Bristol
Silverstone T, Turner P 1982 Drug treatment in
    psychiatry 3rd edn. Routledge & Kegan Paul,
    London

334   It is a procedure whereby a particular behaviour is increased or decreased in frequency by respectively supplying or withholding reinforcement when the behaviour occurs. A reinforcer, either positive or negative, increases the likelihood of the recurrence of a particular behaviour. Positive reinforcers which are perceived as rewards, such as money, praise or cigarettes, follow the response. A negative reinforcer is something unpleasant which ceases when the response is made. Intermittent reinforcement makes the conditioning more resistant to extinction, particularly when a variable schedule of reinforcement is used. Operant conditioning techniques have been applied to a wide range of psychological problems such as stuttering, drug and alcohol abuse, hysterical blindness, anorexia nervosa, classroom behaviour, asthmatic attacks and low back pain. It has been used extensively in the management of the problems of long term hospitalised patients such as those with schizophrenia and mental handicap.

These techniques are also used for patients with chronic physical illness, particularly pain. Biofeedback training involves the principles of operant conditioning.

Atkinson R, Atkinson R, Hilgard E (eds) 1983
   Introduction to Psychotherapy 8th edn. International
   edition. Harcourt Brace Jovanovich, New York
Cobb J 1986 Behavioural psychotherapy. In: Hill P,
   Murray R, Thorley A (eds) Essentials of
   Postgraduate Psychiatry 2nd edn. Grune and
   Stratton, London

335 Briquet, in 1859, noticed a clustering of certain symptoms when describing hysterics and following recent work by psychiatrists in St. Louis, USA, the term 'Briquet's syndrome' has been adopted to encompass these features. So far it has only been described in women and is characterised by longstanding multiple somatic complaints, sexual and gynaecological symptoms and frequent hospitalisations and operations before the age of 30. A tendency to be manipulative with their doctors and a refusal to accept a psychological explanation for symptoms has been described. Premorbid personality traits are frequently noted to be histrionic, but not invariably so and conversion and dissociative features are not a necessary part of the syndrome. The prevalence of the syndrome is estimated to be 1–2% in women and it has been reported to be a familial disorder occurring in 20% of first degree relatives. The features of this syndrome share many of the characteristics of hypochondriacal neurosis, hysterical personality and Munchausen's syndrome and its validity has not been firmly established.

Lancet 1977 Editorial: Briquet's syndrome or hysteria.
   Lancet i: 1138–1139
Perley M J, Guze S B 1962 Hysteria: The stability
   and usefulness of clinical criteria. New England
   Journal of Medicine 266: 421–426

336 A multitude of organic illnesses may produce global intellectual impairment and the cerebral effects of some are reversible if they are correctly diagnosed and given early treatment. Depression may present as a dementing-like illness and may be appropriately treated with tricyclic antidepressants. A large number of metabolic and toxic disorders such as hypothyroidism, hypocalaemia, hypercalcaemia, hypoglycaemia, alcohol depen-

dence and heavy metal poisoning can present as dementia and if they are detected at an early stage their cerebral effect can be interrupted and reversed. The same principles apply to overt and latent renal and hepatocellular failure. The chronic intellectual deterioration which may be associated with a subdural haematoma is another treatable form of dementia. Likewise, infections such as encephalitis, meningitis and neurosyphilis, chronic drug intoxication, chiefly barbiturates and alcohol, pernicious anaemia, resectable tumours and some longstanding cases of epilepsy may all present as dementias which are potentially reversible. The dementing features of normal pressure hydrocephalus may be remarkably improved by a ventriculo–atrial shunt.

Isaacs A 1983 The senium. In: Lader M (ed) Handbook of Psychiatry 2. Mental disorders and somatic illness. Cambridge University Press, Cambridge
Mulley G P 1986 Differential diagnosis of dementia. British Medical Journal 292 (6533): 1416–1419

337 Symmetrical lesions are found constantly in the mamillary bodies and they also occur in the walls of the third ventricle, peri-aqueductal grey matter, floor of the fourth ventricle, the terminal portion of the fornices, the brain stem and in the anterior lobe and superior vermis of the cerebellum. Lesions of the third and sixth nerve nuclei and of the vestibular nuclei are associated with the ocular palsies and nystagmus. The distribution of the lesions are similar in Korsakoff's and Wernicke's syndromes apart from the medial dorsal nucleus of the thalamus and the pulvinar. Lesions in these structures were not demonstrated in patients with Wernicke's syndrome without amnesia and were constantly associated with the Korsakoff's syndrome. These findings might indicate that thalamic lesions are crucial for the development of the amnesic state. Microscopically there are varying degrees of nerve cell loss with astrocytic and microglial proliferation, congestion of blood vessels with or without haemorrhages and endothelial proliferation. Patients with Korsakoff's syndrome show more chronic glial and vascular reactions.

Horel J A 1978 The neuro anatomy of amnesia. A critique of the hippocampal memory hypothesis. Brain 101: 403–445

Victor M 1983 Mental disorders due to alcoholism.
In: Lader M (ed) Handbook of Psychiatry 2 Mental
disorders and somatic illness. Cambridge University
Press, Cambridge

338 The first step would be to assess the risk to the
accused partner. Morbid jealousy is a serious
disorder in that it almost always results in
constant harrassment of the marital partner,
sometimes to the extent that they become clinically depressed or anxious. The possibility that
the jealous partner may resort to murdering the
spouse or the alleged lover must be carefully
considered as it is a very real risk. In the worst
instances compulsory admission to hospital may
be necessary. Where the jealousy is an extension
of the patient's personality or is related to a
change in the patients life circumstances, treatment with a phenothiazine will usually lessen the
intensity of the delusion. However, treatment will
need to be continued as the symptom usually re-
emerges when the medication is stopped. It is also
worthwhile exploring the psychodynamics involved,
particularly where the jealousy is a reaction to an
upset in the patient's life. For example a man who
is impotent may blame his wife's alleged infidelity
for his sexual inadequacy. Jealousy occurring in
association with another psychotic illness usually
remits when the illness abates, but in some
instances the morbid jealousy may become more
apparent and require treatment in its own right.

Shepherd M 1974 Morbid jealousy: A psychiatric
symptom. In: Barraclough B, Heine B, Smith A
(eds) A compilation of papers for the use of
postgraduate students of psychiatry. John Wyeth and
Brothers Ltd, Maidenhead

339 This is a clinical neurological test which is useful
for distinguishing between organic and functional
psychiatric disorders. When light touch stimuli
are applied simultaneously to the cheek and hand,
patients with brain damage often only feel one of
the stimuli or mislocate the more peripheral of the
stimuli. Unlike a focal parietal lobe lesion, the
extinction is present on both sides of the body.
Normal subjects and patients with functional
disorders might not detect or may mislocate one
of the stimuli on the first few trials, but after 10
attempts almost all will be able to distinguish
correctly between the stimuli, while 90% of

patients with brain damage will continue to make errors of extinction or displacement.

Irving G, Robinson R A, McAdam W 1970 The validity of some cognitive tests in the diagnosis of dementia. British Journal of Psychiatry 117: 149–156

340 Hysterical personality disorder can be distinguished and can exist independently of hysteria. Various studies indicate that between 12 and 21% of subjects with hysterical neurosis have a hysterical personality. The personality profile is characterised by a need to influence and please others, a tendency to crave attention and by insincerity and excessive displays of emotion and these traits are enduring. The subjects tend to be exploitive and want to create effect in their manner, speech and dress to the extent of even being theatrical. They crave, in the words of Karl Jaspers, to appear to themselves and to others more than they are, and to experience more than they are capable of. They lack a central core and live behind a series of masks. Lying is often resorted to in an effort to maintain the facade and to impress others. Women with this personality profile are frequently sexually timid, although they may behave and dress in a seductive manner. Many clinicians have emphasised their tendency to be dependant. Hysterical neurosis refers to the symptom cluster that occurs in an attempt to dissociate from a particular feeling or event and may take the form of a dissociative state or conversion reaction. The former may affect memory, consciousness and intellect and the latter may affect mobility and perception and produce blindness, deafness, paralysis or anaesthesia.

Reid R L 1976 Hysteria. In: Silverstone T, Barraclough B (eds) Contemporary Psychiatry. Headley Brothers Ashford, Kent

Walton H J, Presly A S 1973 Use a category system in the diagnosis of abnormal personality. British Journal of Psychiatry 122: 259–269

341 Surveys have indicated that middle aged women are more prone to depression; Skegg and co-workers found that some two-third of consultations for psychiatric symptoms in general practice involve middle age women and about one-third of women aged forty-nine to fifty-nine are likely to receive psychotropics in the course of one year.

However, it is uncertain how relevant the menopausal hormonal changes are, as in these surveys most psychiatric morbidity occurred in women who were menstruating regularly and some studies showed that the rate of psychiatric morbidity was the same in premenopausal, perimenopausal and postmenopausal women, leading some investigators to suggest that there is no evidence that women are at a greater risk of depression during the menopausal years. Furthermore, the association between low plasma oestrogen levels and depression has not been established and replacement oestrogen therapy has no definite effect on depressive symptoms compared to its impact on vasomotor symptoms. It seems more likely that social and psychological factors associated with middle age and the menopause are of aetiological significance. The menopause represents a change of life cycle and for an aging woman whose children are leaving home and whose aging partner may be ill it is a time when her whole direction of life is being questioned.

Osborn M 1984 Depression at the menopause. British Journal of Hospital Medicine 32: 126–129
Skegg D C, Doll R, Perry J 1977 Use of Medicines in General Practice. British Journal of Medicine 1: 1561–1563
Weissman M M, Klerman G L 1977 Sex differences in the epidemiology of depression. Archives of General Psychiatry 34: 98–111

342   The fact that a psychiatrist is asked to assess the degree of dangerousness in an individual before the courts suggest that there is some underlying psychiatric or abnormal explanation for the person's behaviour. This is not necessarily so. The second principle is that the assessment should be objective and this may be particularly difficult if the person has been a patient in the reporting psychiatrist's care for a period of time. It must also be stressed that psychiatrists do not have a foolproof mechanism for predicting dangerousness. The first aspect of the assessment is the analysis of the violent behaviour in terms of its type, frequency, timing, precipitating factors and to ascertain whether there is a mental abnormality or drug or alcohol addiction. Interviews with the patient, relatives and others with whom he has been in contact and information from official criminal records should form the basis of the assessment. The information needs to be inter-

preted in the context of the patient's background, personality, attitudes and mental status. It is important to consider whether there is an underlying problem such as depression, schizophrenia, alcoholism, a neuropsychiatric or medical disorder which may contribute to this behaviour. The model proposed by Megargee whereby violence occurs along a continuum from over-control of impulses with personality rigidity to under-control with habitually aggressive behaviour, although its validity has yet to be confirmed, is considered to be the best model for appraisal of the individual case. Having assessed the possibility of future violent behaviour, the degree of responsibility the person has for his violence needs to be considered and whether he is motivated to change and participate in treatment so that appropriate recommendations on management can be made.

Gunn J 1979 Forensic psychiatry. In:
Granville–Grossman K (ed) Recent Advances in
Clinical Psychiatry 3. Churchill Livingstone,
Edinburgh

343 Bipolar mood disorders tend to run in families in that the risk for a first degree relative having a similar bipolar disorder is 10% and of having a unipolar depression is 11% compared to the average life time risk of 1% for bipolar illness and a prevalence rate for unipolar depression of 3% for men and 6% for women. That this familial tendency is genetic is substantiated by twin and adoption studies: the concordance rate between monozygotic twins with manic-depression is between 60 and 80% compared to a figure of 15 to 20% for dizygotic pairs and the rate of bipolar disorders is significantly higher in the biological than the adoptive parents of manic-depressive patients who were adopted in infancy. These figures are statistical averages and cannot be applied very strictly when giving individual genetic counselling. Recognising that there are diferent treatment responses to lithium and individual antidepressants and that various forms of bipolar illness, such as bipolar I, II and III, have been described suggests that there are different biochemical subtypes of manic-depressive illness, most of which have a mainly genetic basis and others where environmental stresses have a significant aetiological influence. Even within families where there is a very evident familial pattern of mood disorder there is as yet no way of predicting

which offspring are likely to become psychiatrically ill. While genetic counselling need not be postponed until the person has fully adapted psychologically to the implications of the illness, the stages of shock, denial, anxiety, anger and depressions which can precede acceptance need to be given due account.

Nurnberger J I, Gershon E S 1982 Genetics. In: Paykel E S (ed) Handbook of Affective Disorders. Churchill Livingstone, Edinburgh

Pullen I, Emery A 1985 Genetic counselling—A contemporary approach. British Journal of Hospital Medicine 34: 358–360

344 Of all the psychiatric disorders the strongest association is with depression. Gibben and his colleagues found that 10–20% of all women shoplifters had suffered a depression at the time of the original offence. Associated features were medical illness, chronic background difficulties and severe life events. Most of the women were of good previous character and only a small minority had further convictions. It is thought that the unspoken mental distress being experienced at the time becomes expressed as shoplifting and is an unconscious call for help. In other instances the depressed and muddled shopper may unwittingly leave a shop without paying for goods. Patients with alcoholism or schizophrenia may steal out of necessity and for those with mania or anorexia nervosa shoplifting may be a symptom of the disorder. Phobic patients may flee with goods from a crowded shop during a panic attack.

Gelder M, Gath D, Mayou R 1983 Forensic psychiatry, In: Oxford Textbook of Psychiatry. Oxford University Press, Oxford

Gibbens T C N, Palmer C, Prince J 1971 Mental health aspects of shoplifting. British Journal of Medicine iii: 612–615

345 The selection centres on ensuring that the patient's attributes and problems will allow the achievement of the therapeutic goal within the allotted number of therapy sessions. Malan specifically details four stages of selection. The first is the elimination of absolute contraindications such as serious suicidal attempts, chronic drug or alcohol addiction, convinced homosexuality, long term hospitalisation, more than one course of ECT, incapacitating chronic obsessional or phobic symptoms and gross destructive acting

out behaviour. The second aspect of selection is identifying factors which would relatively exclude patients from therapy: an inability to start effective therapeutic work because of an inability to make contact, poor motivation or rigid defences, an inability to terminate because of deep seated problems or severe dependence and a likelihood of developing a depressive or psychotic breakdown. The third aspect of selection is that the therapist must be able to identify a core conflict, focus, or unifying theme and be able to make connections between the past conflicts of childhood, the current conflict brought to therapy and the manifestations of the conflict in the transference. Finally, the patient should be able to think in emotional terms, have the strength and motivation to face disturbing material and be able to respond positively to trial interpretations, based on the focus, given during the assessment period.

Malan D 1976 Selection. In: The Frontier of Brief Psychotherapy. Plenum, New York
Wolberg L R 1977 Short-term psychotherapy. In: The Technique of Psychotherapy 3rd edn. Part II. Grune and Stratton, New York

346 Combined administration of MAOIs and tricyclic antidepressants of the imipramine group will induce a hypertensive crisis. Patients taking clomipramine, imipramine, or other members of this group should not be commenced on a MAOI within fourteen days of discontinuation of the tricyclic. The converse also applies: patients on an MAOI should have their treatment stopped fourteen days before starting a tricyclic of the imipramine group. Amitriptyline, trimipramine and maprotiline are known not to produce hypertensive reactions when combined with a MAOI, but it is usually recommended that the particular tricyclic be prescribed first. Side effects of the tricyclics, such as dry mouth, constipation and postural hypotension are frequently exacerbated by the addition of an MAOI. Phenothiazines, benzodiazepines and lithium can be prescribed with MAOIs, without the risk of producing severe interactions. There is some evidence to suggest that carbamazepine, which has a tricyclic structure, when administered with an MAOI will cause a hypertensive crisis.

Dally P, Connolly J 1981 Psychotropic drugs. In: An Introduction to Physical Methods of Treatment in Psychiatry 6th edn. Churchill Livingstone, London

347 The tremor, which is usually fine, is generally confined to the hands, but may also be seen in the jaw and lower limbs and worsens in anxiety provoking situations. It tends to be more extensive and is more frequently encountered in patients with a family history of essential tremor. The tremor is otherwise related to the concentration of serum lithium. A fine tremor is frequently reported by patients with a serum lithium level within the therapeutic range, but this does not usually require treatment unless it is interfering with manual dexterity or is causing embarrassment. In such instances a slight reduction in the serum lithium concentration will usually lessen the tremor, but this benefit needs to be weighed against the risk of precipitating a relapse of the affective disorder, which can occur with a lithium concentration at the lower end of the therapeutic range. If attempts at reducing lithium dosage are unsuccessful the usual practise is to prescribe propranolol 20–80 mgs. daily in divided doses. A coarse tremor is indicative of neurotoxicity and the serum lithium concentration should be measured immediately. Treatment should be suspended until the tremor has been treated and the reason for the increased serum lithium has been established.

Tyrer S, Shopsin B 1980 Neural and neuromuscular side effects of Lithium. In: Johnson F N (ed) Handbook of Lithium Therapy. MTP Press, Lancaster

348 'Masked' depression indicates that the depressive disorder is presenting in an atypical manner in that the depressive features are not very conspicuous. While there are differences between the various definitions of masked depression, it is probably best considered to occur in three different but somewhat overlapping forms. The first is where a particular depression related symptom such as fatigue or anxiety dominates the clinical picture and depression or feelings of sadness are not very evident. The next group refers to syndromes that present as some physical or non-affective psychiatric disorder such as facial pain, psychosomatic disorder, pseudodementia or hysterical conversion syndrome. The third form refers to those who present with a complication of depression such as alcohol dependence, marital disharmony, shoplifting or exhibitionism.

Bhanji S 1979 Affective disorder. In: Hill P, Murray
R, Thorley A (eds) Essentials of Postgraduate
Psychiatry. Academic Press, London

349 Delinquency tends to run in families; surveys
indicate that juvenile delinquents are twice as
likely to have criminal fathers and where both
parents have criminal records some two-thirds of
the sons will have similar behavioural patterns.
However, in most instances of familial criminal
behaviour the parents are not actively involved in
crime during their children's formative years.
Poor parenting in the form of lax supervision,
excessively indulgent or strict discipline with
inconsistent punishment have been noted in these
families along with family discord. Transmission
of permissive attitudes is also considered to be a
significant formative factor. Although twin studies
indicate a higher concordance rate for monozygotic twins than dizygotic pairs for adult criminality this does not apply to juvenile delinquents.
Juvenile delinquency was once associated with
urban areas of deprivation and was thought to be
a type of behaviour sanctioned by a particular
culture but more recent surveys indicate that it is
more evenly distributed among the social classes.
The varying levels of delinquency that may exist
both between boroughs and streets has been
explained by the contribution of delinquent
families and individual schools.

Hill P 1979 Forensic psychiatry. In: Hill P, Murray
R, Thorley A (eds) Essentials of Postgraduate
Psychiatry 1st edn. Academic Press, London
Power M J, Benn R T, Morris J N 1972
Neighbourhood schools and juveniles before the
courts. British Journal of Criminology 12: 111–132

350 In separate interviews with the child and parents
one would look for a discrepant or vague history
of injury, a delay in reporting injury, or a history
of other children within the family being
subjected to non-accidental injury. Typical
injuries of baby battering include multiple bruises
of varying ages, lacerations of the inner aspect of
the upper lip, multiple fractures, subperiosteal
haematomas, epiphyseal separations, subdural
haematomas and retinal injury. If the cause of the
injuries are not admitted to by the parents and
there is a strong suspicion that the injuries are of

a non-accidental origin then the child must be separated from the parents either with their consent or by a Place of Safety Order pending further assessment. A key worker must be appointed to manage the situation and a surveillance network established to monitor progress. The child's name should be entered on an 'at risk' register if one is available in the area. Assessment of the situation may indicate that the child cannot return home and a Care Order will have to be sought. If the child is returning home the parents' unrealistic expectation of the child will need to be modified and they will require the practical support of facilities such as day nursery and psychotherapeutic help to cope with any personal or marital problems that might exist.

Cameron J M 1970 The battered baby. British Journal of Hospital Medicine 4: 769–778

Hill P 1979 Forensic psychiatry. In: Hill P, Murray R, Thorley A (eds) Essentials of Postgraduate Psychiatry 1st edn. Academic Press, London

351 Clomipramine is claimed to be superior to other antidepressant medication in the treatment of obsessional neurosis. Marks and his colleagues have reported that obsessional neurosis accompanied by varying degrees of depression responded to clomipramine. However, it is not yet clear whether the effect is primarily antidepressive or antiobsessive, although a study by Montgomery and his colleagues found it to be equally effective in obsessive compulsive neurosis, irrespective of the degree of depression. There have been few studies which have compared clomipramine with other tricyclic antidepressants, but there is one report which indicates that clomipramine is superior. Many clinicians have noted that clomipramine is particularly effective for bipolar depression and it is likely that certain biochemical subtypes of depression will only respond to this antidepressant.

Insel T R, Mueller E A 1984 The psychopharmacologic treatment of obsessive-compulsive disorder. In: Insel T R (ed) New Findings in Obsessive Compulsive Disorder. American Psychiatric Press Inc, Washington

Montgomery S 1982 Antidepressant drugs. In: Granville–Grossman K (ed) Recent Advances in Clinical Psychiatry 4(11). Churchill Livingstone, Edinburgh

352   Reports from various treatment centres indicate
       that 20–50% of bipolar patients fail to respond
       prophylactically to lithium. The response rate
       depends on the subtypes being treated; the more
       specialised the unit the more likely it is that it will
       have been referred treatment resistant cases.
       Kukopulous reports that 60–70% of those with a
       mania—depression—interval course of either
       bipolar I or bipolar II pattern respond favourably
       while another 20% have a partial response in that
       the duration and intensity of the depression or
       elation is attenuated. In his series, 20% failed to
       show any prophylactic response and this group
       was mainly comprised of patients with continuous
       cycles and bipolar I patients with a depression—
       mania—interval course. Lithium is an effective
       antimanic agent in 70–80% of cases and there is
       evidence to suggest that responders are more
       likely to have typical manic symptoms without
       schizophreniform features, to have a family
       history of manic-depression and to have intervals
       of significant remissions. Lithium has been advo-
       cated for the treatment of acute depression,
       especially for those with a bipolar pattern, but
       there is little evidence to indicate that it is su-
       perior to tricyclic antidepressants.

       Kukopulous A, Reginaldi D 1980 Recurrence of
          manic-depressive episodes during lithium treatment.
          In: Johnson F N (ed) Handbook of Affective
          Disorders, MTP Press, Lancaster
       Prien R F, Coffey E M, Klett C J 1974 Factors
          associated with treatment success in lithium
          carbonate prophylaxis. Archives of General
          Psychiatry 31: 189–192

353   They are distinguished from normal fears in that
       they are associated with a disproportionate invol-
       untary fear which cannot be explained by the
       particular context and they lead to avoidance of
       a situation or object. Phobic symptoms are
       distinguished from phobic disorders in that they
       occur as part of another psychiatric disorder such
       as depression, obsessional neurosis, generalised
       anxiety neurosis or schizophrenia. Marks has
       distinguished two forms of phobic neurosis, one
       being based on a phobia of external stimuli of
       which agoraphobia, social phobia, blood, injury,
       animal and other specific phobias are examples
       and phobias of internal stimuli such as illness and
       obsessional phobias. Patients with illness phobias

have intense ruminations about illness or death, quite like those of an obsessional disorder, but they are not considered to have the subjective sense of resistance associated with obsessions. The nature of the relationship between phobias of internal stimuli, obsessions and depressive illness and how they should be classified is as yet unclear.

Marks I M 1969 Fears and Phobias. Heinemann, London

Marks I M 1970 The classification of phobic disorders. British Journal of Psychiatry 116: 379–380

354 It is a form of psychotherapy which was developed by Eric Berne to simplify the complex traditional psychoanalytical approach and to present a therapy in simple format so that it would be understood by the layman. He postulated that the human personality is composed of three 'ego states' which are coherent organisations of intellect and emotions. The 'parent ego state' consists of introjected parental valves and admonitions, the 'adult ego state' is that aspect of personality which objectively evaluates the demands of the environment and the 'child ego state' is the spontaneous childlike component of the personality. Communication between individuals' corresponding ego states, for example adult to adult ego state, are called complementary transactions and these can continue indefinitely. A crossed transaction occurs when an ego state, other than the one communicated to, replies and this leads to an abrupt ending of the communication. 'Games' between individuals are forms of overt and covert transactions which produce good or bad feelings in the participants. In the initial interview the transactional therapist tries to understand the client's 'lifescript', the preconscious organisation of his life, laid down in childhood and which dictates how he will feel about himself and how he will interact with others. There are four forms of life script: I'm okay—You're okay, I'm not okay—You're okay, I'm not okay—You're not okay and I'm okay—You're not okay. Therapy involves understanding the client's lifescript, pointing out the role of the ego states in communication and encouraging the client after the development of rapport to construct a new reality orientated lifescript.

Berne E 1964 Games People Play. Grove Press, New York

James M, Jongeward D 1971 Born to win:
  Transactional analysis with Gestalt Experiments.
  Addison Wesley, Reading, Massachuttes

355   A strongly held obsession which is not regarded
as being senseless and is not resisted by the
patient can be indistinguishable from a delusion.
Obsessions are however regarded as being the
patient's own thoughts and they are perceived as
persisting without cause. Some clinicians regard
obsessive compulsive neurosis as a variant or
precursor of schizophrenia. However, most
studies indicate that the incidence of schizophrenia among the first degree relatives of obsessive compulsive patients is no higher than in the
general population. Follow-up studies of obsessive
compulsive patients show that no more than 3%
develop schizophrenia. A large retrospective
survey conducted by Rosen found that 3.5% of
schizophrenics had obsessional symptoms and in
every case the obsessional features had preceded
or accompanied the emergence of the schizophrenic symptoms. Those who had preceding
obsessional symptoms tend to develop less severe
personality disintegration, particularly when the
obsessions had predated the psychosis by years.
The association between schizophrenia and
obsessive compulsive neurosis would appear to be
tenuous, if one exists at all.

Black A 1974 The natural history of obsessional
  neurosis. In: Beech H R (ed) Obsessional States.
  Methuen, London
Rosen I 1957 The clinical significance of obsessions
  in schizophrenia. Journal of Mental Science
  103: 773–785

356   A woman who kills her child within a year of its
birth may enter a defence of infanticide. This
allows a reduction of the charge from one of
murder, which carries an automatic sentence, to
one of manslaughter. The defence has to show
that the woman was psychiatrically disturbed
leading to an alteration in the balance of her mind
by the effect of giving birth or subsequent
lactation.

Gunn J 1979 Forensic psychiatry. In:
  Granville–Grossman K (ed) Recent Advances in
  Clinical Psychiatry 3. Churchill Livingstone,
  Edinburgh
Hill P 1979 Forensic psychiatry. In: Hill P, Murray
  R, Thorley A (eds) Essentials of Postgraduate
  Psychiatry (16) 1st edn. Academic Press, London

357 Recent twin studies suggest that there is an important genetic component in phobic disorders. Carey found that there was a higher concordance among monozygotic twins (MZ) than dizygotic twins (DZ) for phobic symptoms but not for the diagnosis of phobic disorders. Torgersen found that MZ pairs were more similar than DZ twins for the strength and type of phobia, except for agoraphobia. While there is a tendency for fear to run in families it is likely that the effect of learned behaviour and modelling contribute significantly to familiality. The onset of a phobia is frequently related to a traumatic event and once an avoidance pattern of behaviour is adopted the phobia is maintained by a form of operant conditioning. There is an association between agoraphobia and a childhood history of separation anxiety. Certain phobias such as agoraphobia, social and illness phobias are related to mood and anxiety disturbances. Another probable contributor to the development of phobias is the human phylogenetic predisposition to learn certain stimulus-response links for height and specific animals. Psychoanalysts maintain that phobics have an inner repressed mental conflict and that the feared object is merely a symbol for more fundamental and hidden fears.

Carey G, Gottesman I 1981 Twin and family studies of anxiety phobic and obsessive disorders. In: Klein D F, Radkin J G (eds) Anxiety: New Research and Changing Concepts. Raven Press, New York

Marks I M 1969 Fears and Phobias. Heinemann, London

Torgersen S 1983 Genetic factors in anxiety disorders. Archives of General Psychiatry 40: 1085–1089

358 Resistances occur in a variety of subtle and complex ways, in combinations or in mixed forms and single, isolated examples are not the rule. It presents in many guises and can often conceal itself from experienced therapists. Typical examples are where the patient wastes time with small talk, comes late for sessions, has prolonged silences, complains repeatedly about symptoms, acts out, dissociates the therapy sessions from his everyday life, is unable to think or to feel, makes self derogatory remarks to underline their inability to change their life or regards the therapy sessions as almost always being cheerful hours. Intellectual insight is another form of resistance, where the

patient can give a clear account of the psychodynamics but continues to behave in his usual manner. Reluctance to give up the pleasurable experience of the therapy and transference reactions are other forms of resistance.

Greenson R R 1967 Resistance. In: The Technique and Practice of Psychoanalysis Part I. International University Press, New York

Wolberg L R 1977 The handling of resistances to cure. In: The Technique of Psychotherapy, PART II 3rd edn. Grune and Stratton, New York

359 Obsessions are recurring unwanted thoughts, ideas, images or impulses that invade a person's consciousness, evoke anxiety or distress and on quiet reflection are regarded as being senseless. While Kurt Schneider's description of obsessive-compulsive phenomena emphasised the subjective feeling of how senseless the obsessions are and how the compulsions are always resisted by the patient, more recent work has shown that a quarter of patients do not consider their obsessions to be senseless and only about a half show more than slight resistance to carrying out the rituals. Compulsions are repetitive behaviours following on an obsession, they are accompanied by a sense of subjective compulsion and they aim to produce or prevent some future event or situation. Obsessions and compulsions can, however, run independent courses, even when the same patient has both phenomena. Compulsions can occur in the apparent absence of an obsession, especially where the problem is primary obsessional slowness, but they can also occur alone in compulsive hand washing. Obsessions often persist without translation into any overt activity.

Black A 1974 The natural history of obsessional neurosis. In: Beech H R (ed) Obsessional States. Methuen, London

Stern R S, Cobb J P 1978 Phenomenology of obsessive-compulsive neurosis. British Journal of Psychiatry 132: 233–239

360 There have been few controlled follow-up studies of phobias so that little is known about their natural history. Agras and colleagues carried out a five year follow-up study and found that childhood phobias had improved or remitted at five years, but that the prognosis for the adult form was less favourable. The rate of improvement for

adult phobias of 43% was the same for the treated and untreated group. Animal and specific situational phobias show a better response to treatment than social phobia and agoraphobia. While agoraphobia does respond to behaviour therapy the symptom relief is often incomplete. Some more recent studies indicate that almost three-quarters of agoraphobics who initially responded to treatment remained well at five to nine years follow-up.

Agras W S, Chapin H N, Oliveau D 1972 The natural history of phobias. Archives of General Psychiatry 26: 315–317

Munby M, Johnston D W 1980 Agoraphobia: The long term follow-up of behavioural treatment. British Journal of Psychiatry, 137: 418–427

361 The principal characteristics are that these individuals are solitary, detached and remain distant from others. They have few friends, are usually described as being quiet, emotionally cold and shy and these features are present from early childhood. Instead of being involved with people centred activities, they are more likely to pursue interests such as engineering and science. The schizoid personality can retain an active emotional life through diary keeping and day dreaming. In childhood, because of their shyness, they are often made fun of by their peers and in adult life they find it hard to work as part of a team. They tend to be mistrustful of others, tend to see slights where none is intended and they find it difficult to empathise or understand others motives. When stressed they will tend to retain control by being rigid and determined.

Mann A H, Jenkins R, Cutting J, Cowen P J 1981 The development and use of a standardised assessment of abnormal personality. Psychological Medicine 11: 839–847

Walton H J, Presly A A 1973 Use of a category system in the diagnosis of abnormal personality. British Journal of Psychiatry 122: 259–269

362 Pilowsky conducted a factor analysis of symptoms reported by patients with hypochondriacal complaints and identified three factors: bodily preoccupation, morbid fear of disease and a conviction of the presence of disease which is unresponsive to reassurance. There is considerable doubt about the existence of hypochondriasis as

a primary disorder and hypochondriacal symptoms are most frequently encountered in connection with other disorders such as depressive, anxiety, phobic and obsessive compulsive states. The over-valued ideas of bodily concern may become delusional in depressive and schizophrenic disorders. Kenyon has proposed that hypochondriasis should be considered in the framework of a continuum of increasing concern with health beginning with an over-awareness of normal bodily sensations passing to mild apprehension, phobic concern, over-valued ideas and then to a delusional conviction of the presence of disease. Whether a person responds to a noxious internal stimulus depends on their learned perception of such stimuli and the degree of interoceptive focusing which in turn is influenced by anxiety and depression and it may be constitutionally determined. It is patients with the constitutional predisposition that are thought to develop primary hypochondriasis and have hypochondiracal personalities. Primary hypochondriasis, if it exists, is a rare disorder which is inclined to present as a chronic monosymptomatic somatic complaint in the absence of an affective disorder, schizophrenia, cerebral organic disorder or conversion hysteria. Hypochondriacal personalities are subjects who may have food fads, are overly concerned with physical fitness and bowel functions, take excessive steps to avoid disease and attend their doctor with minor complaints.

Kenyon F E 1976 Hypochondriacal states. British Journal of Psychiatry 129: 1–14.

Pilowsky I 1970 Primary and secondary hypochondriasis. Acta Psychiatrica Scandinavica, 46: 273–285

Thorley A 1986 Neurosis and personality disorder. In: Hill P, Murray R, Thorley A (eds) Essentials of Postgraduate Psychiatry 2nd ed. Grune and Stratton, London

363 As a syndrome this refers to a personality profile associated with antisocial conduct which is not due to mental illness proper or mental subnormality. While the description of the personality type has varied according to the theoretical explanations of its aetiology and the way mental disorders are defined, it has still retained the above characteristics. The sociopath or psychopath has a serious defect of feeling in that he cannot

perceive how his behaviour harms others and has a limited ability to learn from his experiences. However, the psychopath does have a conscience and is quick to point out the shortcomings of others. The psychopath is relatively unaffected by setbacks, punishment, or other painful experiences and will tend to repeat the antisocial acts. The sociopath may be superficially engaging but has trouble sustaining satisfactory relationships and thus marital, social and work relationships are frequently in great disarray. Impulsiveness is usually evident and destructive outbursts may occur without adequate provocation. The sociopath will usually have difficulty waiting for gratification, needs instant excitement and in this context will often seek pleasure through alcohol or drugs. Two forms of psychopathy can be identified, the predominantly aggressive destructive type and the passive drifter, and both are best conceptualised along dimensional lines rather than as categories.

Lewis A J 1974 Psychopathic personality: A most elusive category. Psychological Medicine 4: 133–140
Walton H J, Foulds G A, Littman S K, Presley A S 1970 Abnormal Personality. British Journal of Psychiatry116: 497–510

364   Several investigators have reported an excess occurrence of unpleasant life events prior to the onset of obsessive compulsive neurosis and stress is considered to play an important part in the onset of the neurosis in one half to two-thirds of subjects. Patients who have obsessional, sensitive and anxious personality traits develop the neurosis with a minimum of stress while those with robust premorbid traits tend to decompensate into the neurosis only after experiencing a number of negative life events.

McKeon P, Roa B, Mann A 1984 Life events and personality traits in obsessive compulsive neurosis. British Journal of Psychiatry 144: 185–189
Pollitt J 1969 Obsessional states. British Journal of Hospital Medicine, 2: 1146–1150

365   Patients with excessive narcissism have a great need for personal admiration and they tend to conceive therapy as a means of making themselves more worthy of praise. They concentrate most of their interest on themselves and their extremes of self-love may develop into grandiose strivings,

omnipotent impulses and megalomania. Their dress and manner is often out of keeping with the accepted style and their behaviour is generally exhibitionistic. When Freud differentiated the transference neuroses from the narcissistic neuroses he was stressing the fact that patients who developed a transference neurosis were able to form and sustain a cohesive yet multiform and influential set of transference reactions, whereas the latter have only fleeting transference reactions and therefore were inaccessible and unsuitable for psychoanalytic therapy. Patients with marked narcissistic features are not usually motivated for therapy and they are usually in treatment at the behest of others who are concerned about their behaviour. Their grandiose facade conceals a helpless and impoverished self and their limited ego strengths curtail their ability to absorb insights. In recent years interest in the therapy of narcissistic individuals has been revived and attempts have been made to differentiate them from those with schizophrenia and borderline states. All three are thought to have their origins in the primary stages of separation of self from others. Object relationships become distorted and shallow and are orientated around what they can do to enhance their status and interests.

Greenson R R 1967 Transference. In: The Technique and Practice of Psychoanalysis. International University Press, New York

Wolberg L R 1977 Psychotherapy in special conditions. In: The Technique of Psychotherapy Part II, 3rd ed. Grune and Stratton, New York

366 Court statistics indicate that serious offenders who have been convicted of violent crimes, sexual offences and criminal damage including arson are more likely to be sent to hospital than other offenders. Walker and McCabe's survey found that 41% of offenders are diagnosed as having schizophrenia, 35% have subnormal intelligence, 12% are personality disordered, 8% have an affective disorder. Prisoners referred to hospital are only a small proportion of those sentenced. Gunn's survey of south-east English Prisons found that 31% of inmates could be regarded as psychiatric cases and this figure is considerably in excess of the level of psychiatric morbidity in general practise. While any psychiatric disorder can be associated with criminal activity, personality disorder, alcoholism, drug addiction and mental

handicap are the more frequently encountered syndromes and various surveys indicate that 20–40% of prison inmates have psychopathic personalities. Mental handicap is particularly associated with sexual offences, such as indecent exposure, and arson.

Gunn J 1977 Criminal behaviour and mental disorder. British Journal of Psychiatry 130: 317–329
Walker N McCabe S 1973 Crime and insanity in England, 2. Edinburgh University Press, Edinburgh

367 Patients admitted on emergency orders 4, 5, 130 or 136, for 72-hours, can be discharged by the responsible medical officer. Patients on a Section 2 order, that is admitted for up to twenty-eight days of assessment and those admitted on a Section 3 order for up to six months of treatment can be discharged by the responsible medical officer, hospital manager, the nearest relative or a Mental Health Review Tribunal. When a court imposes a hospital order under Section 37, which is for a six months duration, the responsible medical officer can discharge the patient. If, however, an order is also made under Section 41 by a Crown Court the medical officer requires the consent of the Secretary of State for Home Affairs to discharge the patient. A Mental Health Review Tribunal can also order the release. When the Home Secretary authorises the transfer of a prisoner to hospital under Section 47 it becomes a notional Section 37 order once the prisoner has completed his sentence as defined by the court. However, the Home Secretary can make the direction with or without special restrictions regarding discharge under Section 49 and the method of discharge is then the same as that under Sections 37 and 41.

Gelder M, Gath D, Mayou R 1983 Appendix: The law in England and Wales. In: Oxford Textbook of Psychiatry. Oxford University Press, Oxford

368 There is no clearly superior method of management of psychopathic disorder. It is generally agreed that individual psychotherapy is unhelpful and unless some control is exerted by the individual's peers or his environment little change is likely to occur. The most an outpatient counselling service is likely to achieve is to engender insight into the patient and relatives and to limit the distress families will encounter by continuing

to rescue the patient from his misadventures. Small group therapy sessions where all members have antisocial personalities can be helpful in setting limits on behaviour, defining goals and promoting insight. In-patient therapeutic communities such as those at Henderson and Grendon Underwood Prison have achieved a success rate of 40% based on ex-patients being self supporting and not being involved in further criminal activity. In such an in-patient environment patients work and live together and through the medium of regular group meetings they regulate their activities, define their responsibilities and examine the effect of their behaviour on each other. While there have been no control studies of the effect of therapeutic communities, a follow-up survey by Gibbens and his colleagues, which show that 24% cent of psychopaths identified in prison were out of trouble eight years after release, provides a useful comparison.

Craft M, Stephenson G, Granger C 1964 A controlled trial of authoritarian and self-governing regimes with adolescent psychopaths. American Journal of Orthopaedic Psychiatry 34: 543–554

Gibbons T C N, Pond D A, Stafford–Clarke D 1959 A follow-up study of criminal psychopaths. Journal of Mental Science 105: 108–115

Whiteley J S 1970 The Psychopath and his treatment. British Journal of Hospital Medicine 3: 263–270

369   A plea of diminished responsibility is used as a defence only against a charge of murder. A conviction of murder carries an automatic life sentence and a successful defence on the grounds of diminished responsibility results in a verdict of 'guilty of manslaughter' which leaves the sentence to the Judge's discretion. As the McNaughton rules are very restrictive the defence is more likely to enter a plea of diminished responsibility where it is considered that a mental disorder has 'substantially impaired the person's mental responsibilities for his acts and omissions in doing or being a party to the killing'. Successful pleas have been based on grounds of functional and organic psychosis, emotional immaturity, psychopathic personality disorder and premenstrual tension. If the plea is not acceptable to the prosecution, the trial proceeds and the jury decide whether the impairment was sufficient to substantially impair responsibility. Sometimes the McNaughton rules are entered as a defence to

obtain a verdict of 'not guilty', as a conviction of manslaughter is officially registered and will affect employment prospects, insurance and foreign travel.

Gelder M, Gath D, Mayou R 1983 Forensic
    Psychiatry. In: Oxford Textbook of Psychiatry.
    Oxford University Press, Oxford
Gunn J 1979 Forensic Psychiatry, In: Granville-
    Grossman K (ed) Recent Advances in Clinical
    Psychiatry 3. Churchill Livingstone, Edinburgh

370 The more frequently encountered traits are those of excessive cleanliness, orderliness, pedantry, conscientiousness, uncertainty, indecisiveness, rigidity and lack of adaptability. They are relatively enduring characteristics and are considered to be egosyntonic. Obsessional personalities need to be in control and are upset if their routine is disturbed. While the more marked forms of these traits are readily recognisable, more subtle forms may only appear when the person is stressed. Lewis postulated that there were two forms of obsessional personality, one obstinate, morose and irritable, the other vacillating, uncertain and submissive.

Lewis A J 1936 Problems of obsessional illness.
    Proceedings of the Royal Society of Medicine
    29: 325–336
Walton H J, Presly A S 1973 Use of a category system
    in the diagnosis of abnormal personality. British
    Journal of Psychiatry 122: 259–267

371 Current evidence does support the idea of an increased propensity for criminal behaviour in those with the 47 XYY syndrome. Studies indicate that men who are found to have the chromosomal abnormality in general population surveys are more likely to have criminal records and their crimes are likely to be more serious than the average criminal even when factors such as height, intelligence and parental socio-economic status are taken into account. The chromosomal abberation is encountered twenty times more often among the inmates of maximum security institutions for mentally abnormal offenders than it is among new born males. However, not all 47 XYY subjects have criminal tendencies and although those with the disorder who have criminal tendencies are found to be socially deprived, less intelligent, impulsive and immature

what is peculiar to the 47 XYY subject in terms of its association with criminal behaviour is unknown.

Pitcher D C R 1982 Sex chromosome disorder. In: Granville–Grossman K (ed) Recent Advances in Clinical Psychiatry 4. Churchill Livingstone, Edinburgh

Witkin H A, Mednick S A, Schulsinger F, Bakkestrom E, Christiansen K O, Goodenough D R, Hirschhorn K, Lundsteen C, Owen D R, Philip J, Rubin D B, Stocking M 1976 Criminality in XYY and XXY men. Science 193: 547–555

372 This term describes the dissociation of affect which is seen in conversion hysteria. It allows the subjects have severe disabilities and gross symptoms and yet remain detached or undisturbed by their suffering.

Hamilton M 1985 Disorders of emotion. In: Fish's Clinical Psychopathology. Wright, Bristol

373 For a person to make a legally valid will in the presence of a disturbed mental state he must be of sound disposing mind. This means that he must know what a will is, what the extent and nature of his property is, who his close relatives and friends are and who would have a claim on the property. The doctor must ascertain whether the patient's disordered mental state has influenced his feelings or judgement in making the will. A person who is intermittently confused but is judged, on the basis of an interview with a doctor, to know what he is about to do can make a will. Patients who have senile dementia are very suggestible and may mistake a grandson for a son or a housekeeper for a daughter and exclude somebody from their will on an irrational basis. If the will is very complex then it must be ascertained whether he understands the nature of the will in question. The testator should be interviewed alone and the patient's relatives and friends should be interviewed to check the accuracy of the patient's account.

Gelder M, Gath D, Mayou R 1983 Forensic Psychiatry. In: Oxford Textbook of Psychiatry. Oxford University Press, Oxford

374 As this is a form of psychotherapy that aims to produce limited but definite changes in the patient and as it is time limited, the contraindications to its use are the absence of an identifiable focus for

the therapy after the assessment period and the presence of factors such as a history of serious suicidal behaviour, addiction, convinced homosexuality, long term hospitalisation, incapacitating chronic obsessional or phobic symptoms or gross destructive acting out. Patients who find it difficult to make emotional contact, who have extremely rigid defences, limited motivation for change, intense dependency needs or are likely to have an intensification of a depressive or psychotic disturbance are likely to be considered unsuitable for brief psychotherapy. Deep rooted problems which cannot be incorporated into a psychodynamic focus after a few sessions are unlikely to benefit from brief therapy.

Malan D H 1979 Individual psychotherapy and the science of psychodynamics. Butterworth, London

Sifneos P E 1972 Short term psychotherapy and emotional crisis. Harvard University Press, Cambridge, Massachusettes

375 If a person is incapable of managing their affairs because of illness they may sign over power of attorney to someone whom they choose to act on their behalf. The person must be able to understand the nature of what they are doing and can revoke the powers they have granted at anytime. Although it is a relatively simple procedure, if the person is psychiatrically ill they must be of sound disposing mind to convey power of attorney. If the person is not mentally fit to give power of attorney a relative can apply to the Court of Protection in England and Wales or the Court of Session in Scotland where the medical evidence will be assessed and a receiver appointed. The receiver is usually a close relative and the Lord Chancellor also appoints Legal and Medical Lord Chancellor's visitors who monitor how the person's affairs are being managed.

Hill P 1979 Forensic Psychiatry. In: Hill P, Murray R, Thorley P (eds) Essentials of Postgraduate Psychiatry 1st edn. Academic Press, London

Gelder M, Gath D, Mayou R 1983 Forensic Psychiatry. In: Oxford Textbook of Psychiatry. Oxford University Press, Oxford

376 Severe or psychotic post-natal depression has an incidence of about 0.5%, moderate depression an incidence of 12% and some 50% of women get

mild depressive symptoms which last up to a few days. The risk of recurrence for severe episodes is 14 to 20% and it is unrelated to the length of the interval between pregnancies. Relapse rates for milder forms of depression have not been studied. Patients with severe post-natal depression have similar rates of previous psychiatric and family morbidity as those with non-puerperal affective psychosis. Milder reactive-neurotic depressions occurring post-natally are more likely to occur in women who have had similar episodes, both before and during pregnancy. Problematic life events such as having a pre-term baby, being unhappy about the pregnancy and having an unsatisfactory marriage, or other longstanding difficult circumstances have been shown to be factors contributing to the development of reactive-neurotic post-natal syndromes. There appears to be no association between post-natal depression and social class, marital status, age or parity.

Pitt B 1982 Depression and child birth. In: Paykel E S (ed) Handbook of Affective Disorders. Churchill Livingstone, London

Watson J P, Elliot S A, Rugg J A, Brough D I 1984 Psychiatric disorder in pregnancy and the first post-natal year. British Journal of Psychiatry 144: 453–462

377 After achieving the purpose of the therapy, termination is started by discussing with the patient the possibility of ending treatment weeks to months before the final session. During this tapering off period, in which the frequency of sessions can be gradually reduced, the therapist can deal with any resistance to termination that might arise. The therapeutic work at this phase of the therapy with every patient involves analysising the dependency elements in the therapeutic relationship, searching for the needs of the patient to perpetuate the dependency and encouraging the achievement of as much independence and assertiveness as possible. The therapist will usually need to be less directive at this stage of therapy to allow the patient to take complete responsibility for his own decisions. Termination before achieving the therapeutic goal, because of strong countertransference, stubborn resistance or because of the therapist or patient being unable to continue the treatment for practical reasons, will be dictated by the individual circumstances. Abrupt termination

is sometimes necessary and it does not always mean that further improvement will not occur. Patients will often continue to make positive changes in their lives after abrupt terminations for example, where a subtle transference resistance had been hampering progress in therapy. During the termination phase the possibilities of relapses will need to be explained and the patient given the opportunity of returning for further sessions. The patient should be encouraged to apply what has been learnt in therapy in that he should examine tensions, anxieties or irrational impulses in terms of their possible meaning, based on what he knows of his basic neurotic patterns.

Wolberg L R 1977 Technical problems of termination. In: The Technique of Psychotherapy Part II, 3rd edn. Grune and Stratton, New York

378   As lithium has a narrow therapeutic index and has serious toxic effects supervising prophylactic treatment centres on maintaining the serum lithium concentration within its therapeutic range. It is recommended that a serum lithium estimation be performed every six to twelve weeks, depending on the degree of therapeutic compliance and the subject's usual serum lithium level. A serum thyroxine, thyroid stimulating hormone assay, urea, electrolytes, serum creatinine, full blood count and urine examination for protein, casts and sugar should be carried out every six months. A yearly physical examination is to be recommended. Screening on a regular basis for side effects such as tremor, polyuria, weight gain, gastrointestinal upset, memory disturbance and skin lesions and making appropriate adjustment in lithium dosage should improve therapeutic compliance.

Gelder M, Gath D, Mayou R 1983 Drugs and other physical treatments. In: Oxford Textbook of Psychiatry. Oxford University Press, Oxford

379   The concentration of tricyclic drugs in plasma following achievement of a steady state vary as much as forty-fold between individuals given the same oral dose. Earlier reports of a curvilinear relationship between plasma tricyclic levels and therapeutic outcome have been confirmed by more recent studies and they show that patients with moderate levels of nortriptyline are more likely to have a favourable therapeutic response. With

amitriptyline the picture is more complex as it is metabolised to nortriptyline. There appears to be an optimum therapeutic range of plasma concentrations for certain tricyclic antidepressants, a range which is comparatively narrow for drugs such as nortriptyline, amitriptyline and possibly protriptyline. Estimation of plasma levels may be useful in detecting those patients who fail to respond because of low plasma concentrations and for those who have dangerously high levels but there is as yet insufficient evidence to support their general use in clinical practice.

Asberg M, Cronholm B, Sjoqvist F, Tuck D 1971 Relationship between plasma level and therapeutic effect of nortriptyline. British Medical Journal 3: 331–334.

Mindham R H S 1982 Tricyclic antidepressants and amine precursors. In: Paykel E S (ed) Handbook of Affective Disorders. Churchill Livingstone, Edinburgh

Montgomery S 1982 Antidepressant drugs. In: Granville–Grossman, K (ed) Recent Advances in Clinical Psychiatry 4. Churchill Livingstone, Edinburgh

380 Anxiety is a normal experience and it is only when it is experienced more intensely or for a longer period than previously that it is going to become a symptom. Symptoms range from mild apprehension and irritability to inattention, fear of losing control or of impending disaster with feelings of depersonalisation, lightheadedness, paraesthesia, tremor, chest pain and sweating. Anxiety as a symptom is present in practically every psychiatric disorder from phobic neurosis to organic brain syndrome and diagnosing anxiety neurosis means excluding as an explanation every psychiatric or medical disorder with which anxiety is associated. Thyrotoxicosis, phaeochromocytoma, carcinoid syndrome, hypoglycaemia, temporal lobe epilepsy, disorders of the limbic system, paroxysmal atrial tachycardia, withdrawal states, caffeine intoxication and drugs such as amphetamines may produce anxiety symptoms which can mimic anxiety neurosis. Having excluded secondary anxiety it is then worthwhile distinguishing between trait and state anxiety. Trait anxiety refers to a life-long tendency to anxiousness, tension and nervousness while state anxiety arises from stress or conflict and is more likely to occur in those with trait anxiety. In state

anxiety or anxiety neurosis the degree of anxiety should be understandable in the context of the patient's premorbid personality and the threatening life events which are being experienced. Anxiety related symptoms occurring in the absence of adequate stress, particularly in patients over the age of forty who are presenting for the first time, often indicate that there is an underlying depressive disorder.

Snaith P 1980 Anxiety and phobic neurosis. In:
  Clinical Neurosis. Oxford University Press, Oxford
Thorley A 1986 Neurosis and personality disorder.
  In: Hill P, Murray A, Thorley A (eds) Essentials of
  Postgraduate Psychiatry 2nd edn. Grune and
  Stratton, London

381 Lithium side effects can be conveniently divided into initial effects occurring between two hours and five days after the start of treatment, later side effects between five days and six weeks and those associated with maintenance treatment. The initial effects which may be encountered are nausea, abdominal discomfort, loose stool, fine tremor, thirst and polyuria and there is evidence to suggest these effects are related to the rate of rise of the lithium concentration rather than the peak level. Later side effects represent the impact of lithium on muscle and include fatigue, lethargy, muscle weakness, tremor and ECG changes along with polyuria and polydypsia. The side effects of maintenance therapy, where the serum level is within the therapeutic range, are fine hand tremor, polyuria, polydypsia, mild memory impairment, emotional blunting, weight gain, acne, exacerbation of psoriasis, goitre, hypothyroidism, leucocytosis and oedema. These side effects, other than the cutaneous reactions, are related to the serum lithium concentration.

Brown W T 1980 The pattern of lithium side effects.
  In: Johnson E N (ed) Handbook of Lithium
  Therapy. MTP Press, Lancaster

382 While the indications for prescribing monoamineoxidase inhibitors (MAOIs) are imprecise, most clinicians who are familiar with their use find them to be effective for atypical or neurotic depressions with anxiety and phobic symptoms. Dally and Connolly describe such subjects as having few endogenous features, having a tend-

ency to blame others for their plight and typically have initial insomnia and tend to oversleep in the morning. Often these symptoms have been present for years or run a chronic phasic course and the subject's personality is usually described as obsessional, anxious, hardworking, with an 'over-active autonomic nervous system'. MAOIs are of little help for inadequate neurotic personalities. The effectiveness of MAOIs in treating phobic anxiety states is well established, but behaviour therapy is generally considered to be the treatment of first choice. However, they are particularly useful for phobic states, particularly agoraphobia, which have failed to respond to behavioural methods.

Nies A, Robinson D S 1982 Monoamine oxidase inhibitors. In: Paykel E S (ed) Handbook of Affective Disorders. Churchill Livingstone, Edinburgh

Sheehan D V Ballenger J, Jacobsen G 1980 Treatment of endogenous anxiety with phobic, hysterical and hypochondriacal symptoms. Archives of General Psychiatry 37: 51–59

383 Anxiety neurosis, affective disorder or an extra-cerebral disorder, such as thyrotoxicosis, would be the most likely possibilities. A patient who gives a history of previous bouts of anxiety, has an anxious premorbid personality, has recently experienced a stressful life event and whose anxiety symptoms are understandable in the context of these factors is likely to have an anxiety neurosis. Anxiety symptoms presenting for the first time in middle or late life often indicate an underlying depression and features such as a broken sleep pattern, morning worsening of symptoms, psychomotor retardation and weight loss usually indicate that the primary diagnosis is an affective disorder. Thyrotoxicosis, paroxysmal atrial tachycardia, hypoglycaemia, phaeochromocytoma, temporal lobe epilepsy and alcohol and drug withdrawl states often presents with anxiety related symptoms.

Thorley A, Stern R 1979 Neurosis and personality disorder. In: Hill P, Murray R, Thorley A Essentials of Postgraduate Psychiatry. Academic Press, London

Tyrer P J 1982 Anxiety states. In: Paykel E S (ed) Handbook of Affective Disorders. Churchill Livingstone, Edinburgh

384 Survey of general practice attenders indicate that between one-quarter and one-third of all illnesses seen by the GP are in the mental disorder category. About one-third of these have hidden psychiatric morbidity. The majority present with minor psychiatric morbidity and only 4% of those with a primary psychiatric complaint have a severe depression. The GPs initial difficulty is in distinguishing primary psychiatric morbidity with somatic features from organic state with secondary psychiatric symptoms. How the patient perceives and describes his symptoms, what expectations he has of his GP and how aware the doctor is of the different modes of presentation of psychiatric illness will determine the diagnosis. Once it is considered that the symptoms fall within the psychiatric domain the doctor is next faced with the difficulty of distinguishing between anxiety states and depressive disorders before proceeding with treatment. It is frequently impossible to make clearcut distinctions between these syndromes where the symptoms are mild and the GP has to work with a provisional diagnosis.

Goldberg D, Huxley P 1980 Mental Illness in the Community: Pathways to Psychiatric Care. Tavistock, London

Williams P, Clare A 1986 Psychiatry in general practice. In: Hill P, Murray R, Thorley A (eds) Essentials of Postgraduate Psychiatry, 2nd edn. Academic Press, London

385 It is important to emphasise that the treatment will not be effective for at least two weeks after achieving a reasonable therapeutic dose. During that interval while the patient may find that the sedative effect of a tricyclic such as amitriptyline may lessen anxiety and improve sleep, its antidepressant action takes longer. Familiarising the patient with the more common side effects such as drowsiness, dry mouth, blurring of vision, constipation, tremor and postural hypotension will help the patient cope better should these effects occur. Gradually increasing the dosage from 25 mgs. daily to a full therapeutic dose over a period of seven to ten days is usually effective in minimising adverse effects and improving therapeutic compliance among out-patients. If the patient has previously had side effects which resulted in premature termination of treatment or because of advanced age is likely to be unable to

tolerate standard doses, then it is advisable to start with 10 mgs. daily and increase to his tolerance level. The patient should be advised to avoid alcohol and not to drive or engage in other activities which might have serious consequences should they become drowsy or have impaired co-ordination. The importance of not stopping treatment as soon as his mood improves needs to be emphasised. Should the patient forget to take the tablets for more than forty-eight hours then it is necessary to gradually re-introduce the treatment to minimise the occurrence of side effects.

Dally P, Connolly J 1981 Psychotropic drugs. In: An Introduction to Physical Methods of Treatment in Psychiatry. Churchill Livingstone, Edinburgh

Watts C A H 1982 Depression in general practice. In: Paykel E S (ed) Handbook of Affective Disorders. Churchill Livingstone, Edinburgh

386 In this form of goal limited therapy, support is offered by an authority figure to a person during a period of illness, turmoil or temporary decompensation. It aims to restore the person's former coping mechanisms and defences by allowing the person to become temporarily dependant on the therapist. Supportive techniques include providing a warm confiding and strong relationship, allowing a degree of dependance sufficient to bring relief, encouraging the person in a directive manner, giving advice, reassurance and positive feedback, motivating independence where appropriate and using medication and other devices to relieve distress. Independence is encouraged as the acute situation subsides, but for some indefinite support is necessary to encourage them to sustain the best possible adjustment in their particular environment. It is of value for stable mature persons who are overwhelmed by environmental changes, for those going through a psychotic disturbance and those with major personality difficulties and others who are unlikely to benefit from interpretive psychotherapy. While supportive psychotherapy is not insight orientated, when the person experiences a reduction in anxiety and recognises the beneficial ingredients of the supportive relationship they often develop a degree of insight.

Gelder M, Gath D, Mayou R 1983 Psychological treatment. In: Oxford Textbook of Psychiatry. Oxford University Press, Oxford

Stewart R L 1975 Psychoanalysis and psychoanalytic psychotherapy. In: Freedman A M, Kaplan H I, Sadock B J (eds) Comprehensive Textbook of Psychiatry. Williams and Wilkins, Baltimore

387 Warmth, genuineness and empathy are qualities that Carl Rogers considered to be essential personality factors for the competent psychotherapist. While a number of studies have tended to validate the importance of these characteristics, recent reviews have indicated that more rigorous studies of the relationships between the Rogerian triad and therapeutic outcome are equivocal. A study, by Strupp and Hadley, of male university students with minor psychiatric morbidity who were randomly assigned to have psychotherapy for a maximum of 25 hours over four months with either professional therapists or professors selected on the basis of their personal qualities, showed that both treatment groups did equally well and both fared slightly better than controls on a waiting list. However, the relative mildness of the psychiatric morbidity of the patients and the brevity of the therapy means that the findings cannot be generalised to indicate that therapists' personal attributes determine outcome. These and other studies of the personality traits of therapists, of their attributes during therapy and of peer ratings have not elucidated variables which correlate with outcome.

Bloch S 1982 Psychotherapy. In: Granville–Grossman K (ed) Recent Advances in Clinical Psychiatry 4. Churchill Livingstone, Edinburgh

Parloff M B, Washow I E, Wolfe B E 1978 Research on therapist variables in relation to process and outcome. In: Garfield S L, Gergin A E (eds) Handbook of Psychotherapy and Behaviour Change: An Empirical Analysis 2nd edn. Wiley, New York

Strupp H H, Hadley S W 1979 Specific Vs non-specific factors in psychotherapy: A controlled study of outcome. Archives of General Psychiatry 36: 1125–1136

388 A detailed psychiatric and medical history with a full general physical examination is essential. In conversion hysteria there is no muscle wasting, muscle power is variable and passive movement may produce contraction of the antagonistic group of muscles. In forearm paralysis of hysterical origin when the arm is flexed at the elbow in supination and the forearm is then allowed to drop

it falls in the same supine position in which it was held while in both organic paralysis and normal subjects the forearm pronates with the palmar surface of the hand downwards. Where a leg is paralysed the hysterical patient, when asked to sit forward from a recumbent position, will keep both legs on the couch while the normal subject will raise both legs equally and in organic paralysis the affected leg is raised higher. While these clinical observations may be helpful, they are not absolutely reliable and an electromyogram and other investigations may be necessary. Tests should be conducted without reinforcing the conversion symptoms. Identify a precipitating life event during history taking or later with the help of hypnosis or intravenous sodium amytal can help to clarify the diagnosis. Finally, it is worth keeping the diagnosis under active review when it is one of primary hysterical neurosis as some will be found at a later stage to have an organic explanation for the paralysis.

Gray M 1978 Hysterical neurosis. In: Neurosis: A comprehensive and Critical Review. Van Nostrand Reinhold, New York

Snaith R P 1981 Hysteria and hypochondriasis. In: Clinical Neurosis (4). Oxford University Press, Oxford

389 There is no characteristic profile for those committing homicide and the crime usually represents a complex interaction between perpetrator and victim. In Britain where some two-thirds of murders are considered to be 'normal' homicides, that is there is a conviction of murder or common law homicide, the crime tends to be committed by young men of lower socio-economic status, the victim is usually a close family member and the murder seldom occurs in the course of robbery or sexual offence. In this group where the murder occurs against the conscious wish of the perpetrator the murderer is usually found to have an overcontrolled personality, to have a sado-masochistic relationship with the victim and frequently both have been consuming alcohol. Sexual murders may result from panic during the offence or be the sadistic act of a shy person with bizarre fantasies. 'Abnormal' murders refer to insane murder, suicide, infanticide and those where the murderer has diminished responsibility. The most common psychiatric disorder encoun-

tered in 'abnormal murderers' is a depressive illness and others include schizophrenia, personality disorder, morbid jealousy syndrome and alcoholism.

Bluglass R 1979 Psychiatric assessment of homicide.
  British Journal of Hospital Medicine 22: 366–370
Gillies N 1976 Homicide in the West of Scotland.
  British Journal of Psychiatry 128: 105–127
Scott P D 1977 Assessing dangerousness in
  criminals. British Journal of Psychiatry
  131: 219–227

390 The main side effects are related to its anticholinergic effect: dryness of mouth, constipation, retention of urine, sweating, postural hypotension, blurred vision, impotence and delay in reaching orgasm. Tremor is also a problem with high doses. Trimipramine is the most sedative of the tricyclic antidepressants and drowsiness is a common side effect in the first few days of treatment. Trimipramine's effect on the cardiovascular system include tachycardia, reduction in myocardial contractility leading to heart failure in those who are predisposed and ECG changes such as flattening of T-waves, ST depression and prolongation of the QT interval. Weight gain is also a fairly common side effect and seems to be secondary to carbohydrate craving. As with other tricyclics, trimipramine lowers the convulsive threshold and may induce epileptic convulsions. Unpleasant dreams are associated with this tricyclic antidepressant and for the elderly or those with alcohol dependance vivid nightmares can occur.

Dally P, Connolly J 1981 Psychotropic drugs. In: An
  Introduction to the Physical Methods of Treatment
  in Psychiatry. Churchill Livingstone, London
Montgomery S 1982 Antidepressant drugs. In:
  Granville–Grossman K (ed) Recent Advances in
  Clinical Psychiatry, 4. Churchill Livingstone,
  Edinburgh

391 There is conflicting and confusing evidence concerning the teratogenic effect of tricyclic antidepressants but they are generally regarded as being safe during pregnancy. The absence of a teratogenic effect of many tricyclic antidepressants has not been fully established and the detection of such an effect is dependent on individual case reports, animal experimentation and epidemiological studies, the latter not often being as exten-

sive as are necessary to allow firm conclusions to be drawn before the particular drug is marketed. While ideally no drug should be prescribed during pregnancy, or for a woman who is likely to become pregnant, the absence of definite evidence to substantiate a foetal damage effect for tricyclics enables them to be prescribed when there are sufficient clinical indications for their use. Babies born to women on these drugs should be carefully monitored for evidence of withdrawal features.

Ellis C, Fidler J 1982 Drugs during pregnancy: Adverse reactions. British Journal of Hospital Medicine 28: 575–584

McEwan H P 1982 Drugs in pregnancy: Prescribing. British Journal of Hospital Medicine 28: 559–565

392 Countertransference is the therapists reaction to the patient as if the patient were a significant person in the therapists early life. It can be a reaction to explicit communications or manifestations of the transference where it is in a sense a response of one subconscious to another. In other instances the countertransference represents an intrusion of the therapist's world into the therapy in an idiosyncratic manner in response to, for example, the patient's mode of speech or dress. 'A countertransference problem' arises when this action is not recognised by the therapist and it will take the form of being bored by the patient, being late for the sessions, using silence as a weapon, being unnecessarily clever or by being drawn into the person's subconscious world by being unduly harsh or permissive. Becoming aware of the countertransference behaviour is the essence of its management; once the therapist can identify their blind spot they can use it to good effect to help the patient.

Rosser R, Kinston W 1986 Psychotherapy: Individual. In: Hill P, Murray R, Thorley A (eds) Essentials of Postgraduate Psychiatry, 2nd edn. Grune and Stratton, London

393 Studies of the psychological consequences of rape indicate that the responses are akin to those that follow sudden unexpected trauma. During the impact phase the person experiences fright bordering on panic and behaves in a self-preserving manner. After the assault a state of shock usually occurs for days or weeks when they may develop feelings of guilt, self blame or

physical complaints. These symptoms either resolve after days to weeks or symptoms of depression, sleep disturbance, phobias or sexual disorder develop. Nadelson and her colleagues found, in a retrospective study, that 41% were clinically depressed eighteen months after the attack, but it is likely that there is a large bias factor in such a retrospective study. Other follow-up studies noted that after two and a half years fear of being alone and being suspicious of others was present in more than half of the victims. One prospective study found that victims had significantly more depressive symptoms up to four months after the assault and a small number had similar symptoms at one year. Where there are prior psychological problems or there is limited support after the assault or the victim is young or from a lower socio-economic group the reaction can be compounded and the person may develop chronic depressive or psychosomatic symptoms, sexual and rape related phobias, or abuse alcohol or drugs.

Mezey G 1985 Rape: Victimological and Psychiatric Aspects. British Journal of Hospital Medicine 33: 152–158

Nadelson C, Notman M, Zackson H, Gornick J 1982 A follow-up study of rape victims. American Journal of Psychiatry 139: 1266–1270

394 Women of child bearing years who are taking lithium must take adequate contraceptive precautions. An international register of pregnancies exposed to lithium revealed that 11% of infants were congenitally malformed compared with the expected range of 3–7% of babies and there was a marked over-representation of Ebstein's anomaly and other severe malformations of the cardio-vascular system. As this effect occurs during the first twelve weeks of pregnancy, women need to be advised about the teratogenic effect. If there are good clinical reasons, lithium can be prescribed after twelve weeks provided that it can be given in divided doses and that the serum lithium is carefully monitored and kept as low as is therapeutically feasible. There is evidence from animal studies that even brief pulses of lithium toxicity can impair foetal development. Renal clearance of lithium rises gradually after the first trimester by 30–50% and then drops dramatically to the pre-pregnancy rate after delivery. It is

recommended that the fall in serum lithium due to the increased renal clearance should not be compensated for by an increased dosage. Any element of hypothyroidism in the mother is going to be accompanied by goitre and hypothyroidism in the neonate and this can lead to respiratory distress during delivery. Prescribing thyroxine for the mother will prevent this complication. It is recommended that a mother who is taking lithium should not breast feed her baby as lithium in her milk will result in the baby having a serum lithium concentration that is 10–50% of that of her level. In such instances a neonate who is already prone to diarrhoea and vomiting may develop lithium toxicity. While most clinicians will choose between breast feeding and lithium some continue to allow both to proceed until complications occur.

Weinstein M R 1980 Lithium treatment of women during pregnancy and in the post-delivery period. In: Johnson F N (ed) Handbook of Lithium Therapy. MTP Press, Lancaster

395   In the past few years the previously recommended therapeutic range for lithium of 0.7 to 1.2 m.mols/litre has been questioned. This range had been established on an empirical basis in that it was shown to have a prophylactic effect on manic-depressive illness and was relatively free of serious side effects. Hullin and his colleagues reported that serum levels of 0.4 to 0.6 m.mols/litre were just as prophylactically effective in those with bipolar and unipolar depression and produced fewer side effects. However, their findings need to be extensively corroborated before a lower dosage regime can be recommended. There is evidence to suggest that patients who have severe episodes of both depression and mania need serum lithium levels above 0.8 m.mols/litre while those who have rapid cycles or who have a depression—mania—interval course of bipolarity do best with serum levels between 0.4 and 0.8 m.mols/litre. A very small proportion of patients, probably about 1%, tend to remain in protracted depressions even with serum lithium levels below 0.4 m.mols/litre.

Hullin P R, McDonald R, Allsop M N 1975 Further report on prophylactic lithium in recurrent affective disorders. British Journal of Psychiatry 126: 281–284

Kukopulos A, Tando L 1980 Lithium non-
responders and their treatment. In: Johnson FN (ed)
Handbook of Lithium Therapy. MTP Press,
Lancaster

396 The decision of whether to stop the lithium treatment must be based on whether the patient is
having fewer mood swings than before starting
treatment and on whether the patient is having
disabling side effects. If a year after treatment the
frequency of depression and mania is the same as
it was before treatment than it is unlikely that the
patient is benefitting. It is important to know why
the patient wants to interrupt treatment as he may
object to taking 'drugs', miss his 'highs' or find
the side effects intolerable. Often an explanation
of the need for treatment or making efforts to
lessen side effects will improve therapeutic
compliance. If lithium treatment appears to have
interrupted the former bouts of depression and
mania then stopping treatment will probably
result in a relapse; one study showed that 50%
relapsed within six months and a further 30%
within the first year of terminating treatment. In
certain circumstances a patient may have been
prescribed lithium prophylactically after a single
episode of mania because he was at a very critical
stage of his career and a further mood disturbance
would have been a very serious blow. Once the
patient has passed through this critical phase of
life it is usual to stop the treatment having taken
account of ongoing stress factors and family
history of affective illness. It is probably best to
phase out the lithium treatment gradually so that
any tendency to relapse abruptly will be
attenuated.

Baastrup P C, Pulson J C, Schou M, Thomsen K,
Amdisen A 1970 Prophylactic lithium: Double blind
discontinuation in manic-depressive and recurrent
depressive disorders. Lancet ii: 326–330

397 While some psychotherapists regard acting out as
always being detrimental to the therapeutic
process and others see it as invariably serving to
generate insight if dealt with psychodynamically,
most would take an intermediate viewpoint and
consider that it should be managed in accordance
with whether it serves as an obstruction to or as
a prelude to learning. Acting out should always
be brought to the attention of the patient and he
should be encouraged to talk about his feelings

before putting them into action. This will help to forestall the acting out. Interpretations will also help to dissipate the need for the uncharacteristic behaviour. This will involve repeated pointing out of the manifestations of the acting out behaviour, showing how it is a resistance to therapy and making links between transference resistance and fantasies or impulses. A prolonged period of working through may be necessary where acting out is a manifestation of transference and resistance. Should the behaviour persist or be potentially dangerous the therapist should be more direct in his handling of the problem by encouraging the patient to change his behaviour, by increasing the frequency of sessions, threatening to end therapy and in some instances using behaviour therapy or drug treatment. Needless to say, where the acting out is extremely disruptive the therapy has to be abruptly terminated.

Wolberg L R 1977 The handling of resistances to cure. In: The Technique of Psychotherapy Part II, 3rd edn. Grune and Stratton, New York

398 Treatment and management will be determined by the extent of the mania and degree of the patient's understanding of the need for psychiatric intervention. Frequently the patient will not realise that he is elated and will be quite dismissive of any treatment. However, if a symptom which might be complained of, such as insomnia, can be used as the focus for treatment the patient may accept the need for medication. If the patient's behaviour is acutely disturbed and he is unwilling to accept treatment, compulsory admission to hospital will be necessary. In the formality of a GPs surgery or in a hospital emergency room the manic patient is often initially relatively composed and it is quite easy to underestimate the extent of the mood disturbance. While mild to moderate hypomanic states can be treated on an out-patient basis with the assistance of a relative to monitor treatment and report progress, more intense manic states are best treated in hospital. In such an environment the patient will be protected from the worst excesses of his manic behaviour and treatment can be carefully monitored. Treatment of first choice is haloperidol and this should be started in doses of 0.5 to 3 mgs. orally every six to eight hours and increased as necessary until the patient is more tranquil. In more disturbed states intravenous haloperidol will

be required. A sedative phenothiazine may also be helpful, particularly to ensure a good nights sleep. It is probably advisable to administer an anti-cholinergic agent for the first few days of treatment to prevent acute dystonic reactions as such reactions tend to further alienate patients against treatment. Once the level of physical hyperactivity has been brought under control with haloperidol it is worth prescribing lithium as it seems to achieve a quicker and more complete remission. If the patient had been taking lithium before the onset of the manic relapse it is often helpful to increase the serum lithium level to between 0.9 and 1.2 m.mol/l as this concentration has more of an antimanic effect. Previous worries about adverse interactions between lithium and anti-psychotic agents seem to have abated, but it is important that the patient's serum lithium concentration, hydration and physical wellbeing are regularly monitored to prevent neurological sequelae.

Gelder M, Gath D, Mayou R 1983 Affective disorders.
  In: Oxford Textbook of Psychiatry. Oxford
  University Press, Oxford

399 A full psychiatric assessment is essential. While those charged with indecent exposure are nearly always exhibitionists, exposure is often a prelude to other sexual activity. The individual exhibitionist is typically a passive, unassertive, socially gauche person with marked inferiority feelings. However, occasionally the exposure is related to a current life stress, alcohol abuse, mania or schizophrenic thought disorder. A thorough assessment will help identify any potentially remedial features. It allows the development of a personally tailored programme to encourage more socially acceptable sexual activity and an aversive approach for the deviant behaviour. This combined approach appears to be most useful but there have been few studies of the effectiveness of the different treatment regimes. The therapeutic effect of a court appearance is usually marked in that only 10 to 20% are reconvicted for a similar offence.

Jones I H, Frei D 1977 Provoked anxiety as a
  treatment for exhibitionism. British Journal of
  Psychiatry 131: 295–300
Rooth F G 1971 Indecent exposure and
  exhibitionism. British Journal of Hospital Medicine
  6: 521–533